Mycosis Fungoides/Sézary Syndrome

It's easy to get lost in the cancer world

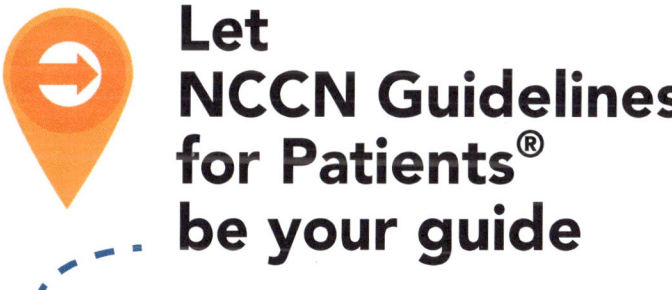

Let NCCN Guidelines for Patients® be your guide

- ✓ Step-by-step guides to the cancer care options likely to have the best results
- ✓ Based on treatment guidelines used by health care providers worldwide
- ✓ Designed to help you discuss cancer treatment with your doctors

About

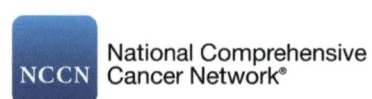

NCCN Guidelines for Patients® are developed by the National Comprehensive Cancer Network® (NCCN®)

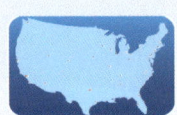

NCCN

- ✓ An alliance of leading cancer centers across the United States devoted to patient care, research, and education

Cancer centers that are part of NCCN:
NCCN.org/cancercenters

NCCN Clinical Practice Guidelines in Oncology (NCCN Guidelines®)

- ✓ Developed by doctors from NCCN cancer centers using the latest research and years of experience
- ✓ For providers of cancer care all over the world
- ✓ Expert recommendations for cancer screening, diagnosis, and treatment

Free online at
NCCN.org/guidelines

NCCN Guidelines for Patients

- ✓ Present information from the NCCN Guidelines in an easy-to-learn format
- ✓ For people with cancer and those who support them
- ✓ Explain the cancer care options likely to have the best results

Free online at
NCCN.org/patientguidelines

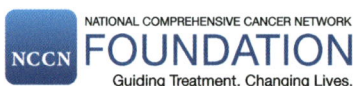

and supported by funding from NCCN Foundation®

These NCCN Guidelines for Patients are based on the NCCN Guidelines® for Primary Cutaneous Lymphomas (Version 1.2021, October 12, 2020).

© 2021 National Comprehensive Cancer Network, Inc. All rights reserved. NCCN Guidelines for Patients and illustrations herein may not be reproduced in any form for any purpose without the express written permission of NCCN. No one, including doctors or patients, may use the NCCN Guidelines for Patients for any commercial purpose and may not claim, represent, or imply that the NCCN Guidelines for Patients that have been modified in any manner are derived from, based on, related to, or arise out of the NCCN Guidelines for Patients. The NCCN Guidelines are a work in progress that may be redefined as often as new significant data become available. NCCN makes no warranties of any kind whatsoever regarding its content, use, or application and disclaims any responsibility for its application or use in any way.

NCCN Foundation seeks to support the millions of patients and their families affected by a cancer diagnosis by funding and distributing NCCN Guidelines for Patients. NCCN Foundation is also committed to advancing cancer treatment by funding the nation's promising doctors at the center of innovation in cancer research. For more details and the full library of patient and caregiver resources, visit NCCN.org/patients.

National Comprehensive Cancer Network (NCCN) and NCCN Foundation, 3025 Chemical Road, Suite 100, Plymouth Meeting, PA 19462
215.690.0300

Supporters

Endorsed by

The Leukemia & Lymphoma Society
The Leukemia & Lymphoma Society (LLS) is dedicated to developing better outcomes for blood cancer patients and their families through research, education, support and advocacy and is happy to have this comprehensive resource available to patients. lls.org/patientsupport

To make a gift or learn more, please visit NCCNFoundation.org/donate or e-mail PatientGuidelines@nccn.org.

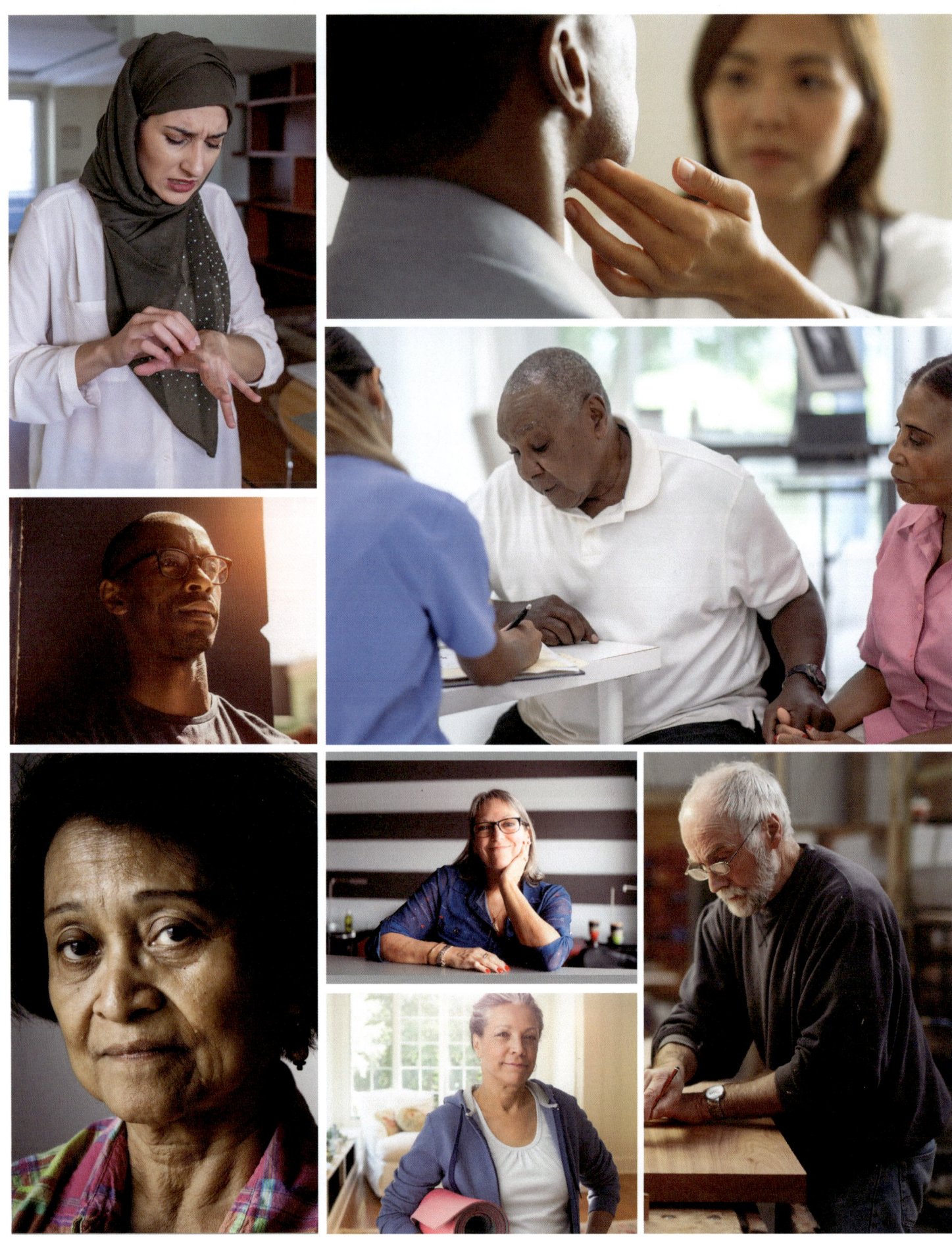

Mycosis Fungoides/Sézary Syndrome

Contents

6 MF/SS basics

13 Testing for MF/SS

30 Treating MF/SS

40 Stage 1A

45 Stage 1B and 2A

51 Stage 2B

56 Stage 3

60 Stage 4

66 Large-cell transformation

70 Making treatment decisions

84 Words to know

86 NCCN Contributors

87 NCCN Cancer Centers

88 Index

1
MF/SS basics

7	The lymphatic system
8	Lymphocytes
9	Cutaneous T-cell lymphoma
10	Mycosis fungoides
11	Sézary syndrome
12	Review

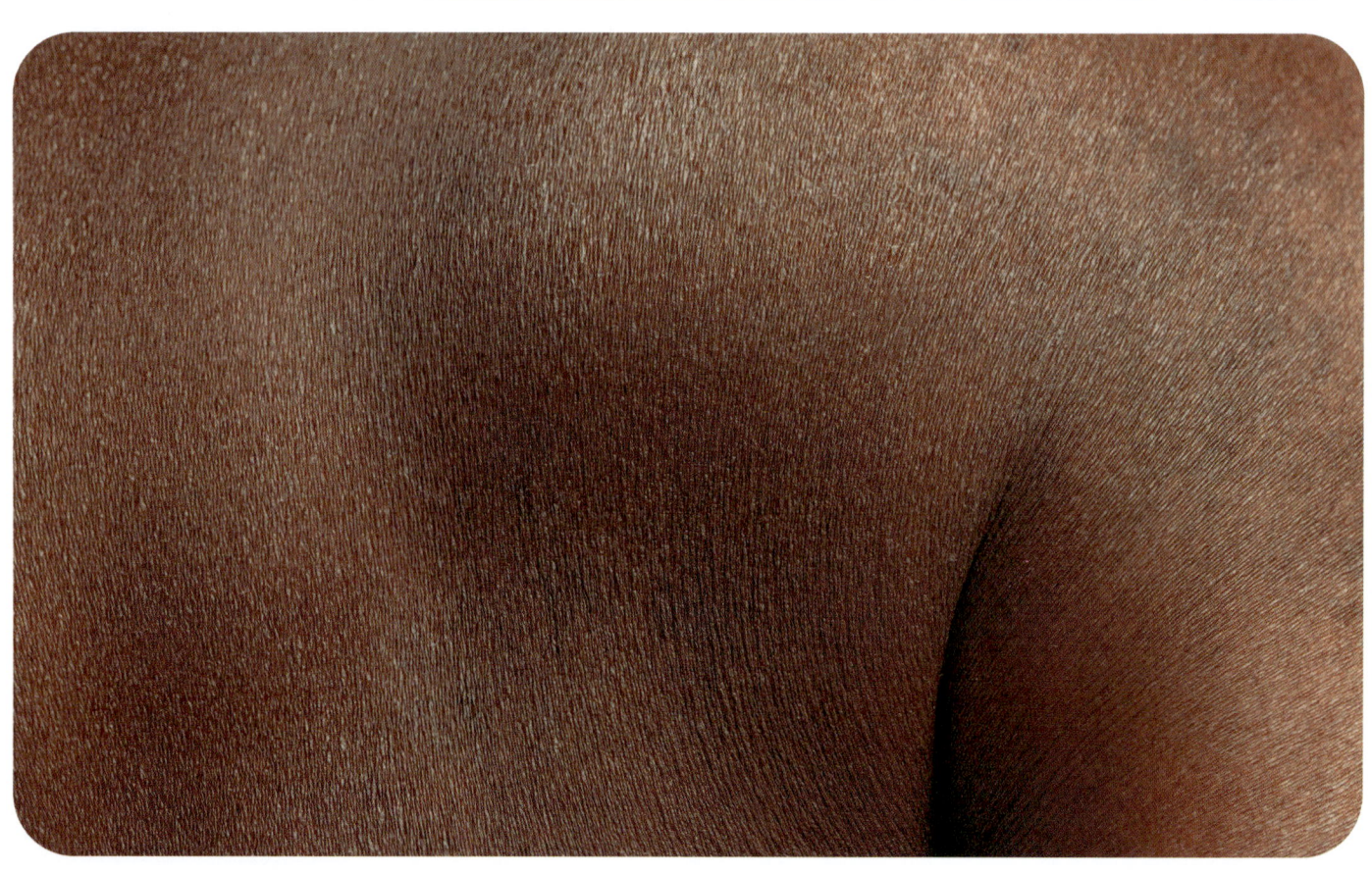

1 MF/SS basics | The lymphatic system

Mycosis fungoides (MF) and Sézary syndrome (SS) are types of skin lymphomas called cutaneous T-cell lymphoma (CTCL). CTCL is a rare form of cancer that develops when your T cells grow abnormally in the skin. These cells can grow in the blood, lymph nodes, or other areas of the body, as well. Although the skin is involved, the skin cells themselves are not cancerous.

The lymphatic system

Lymphoma is the most common type of blood cancer. It affects the lymphatic system. The lymphatic or lymph system is a major part of the body's immune system. It is a germ-fighting network of tissues and organs that includes the bone marrow, spleen, thymus, lymph nodes, and lymphatic vessels.

Lymphatic vessels are a network of thin tubes that carry lymphatic fluid (lymph) and white blood cells into all the tissues of the body. As lymph travels throughout your body, it passes through hundreds of small bean-shaped structures called lymph nodes. Lymph nodes make immune cells that help the body fight infection. They also filter the lymph fluid and remove foreign material such as bacteria and cancer cells.

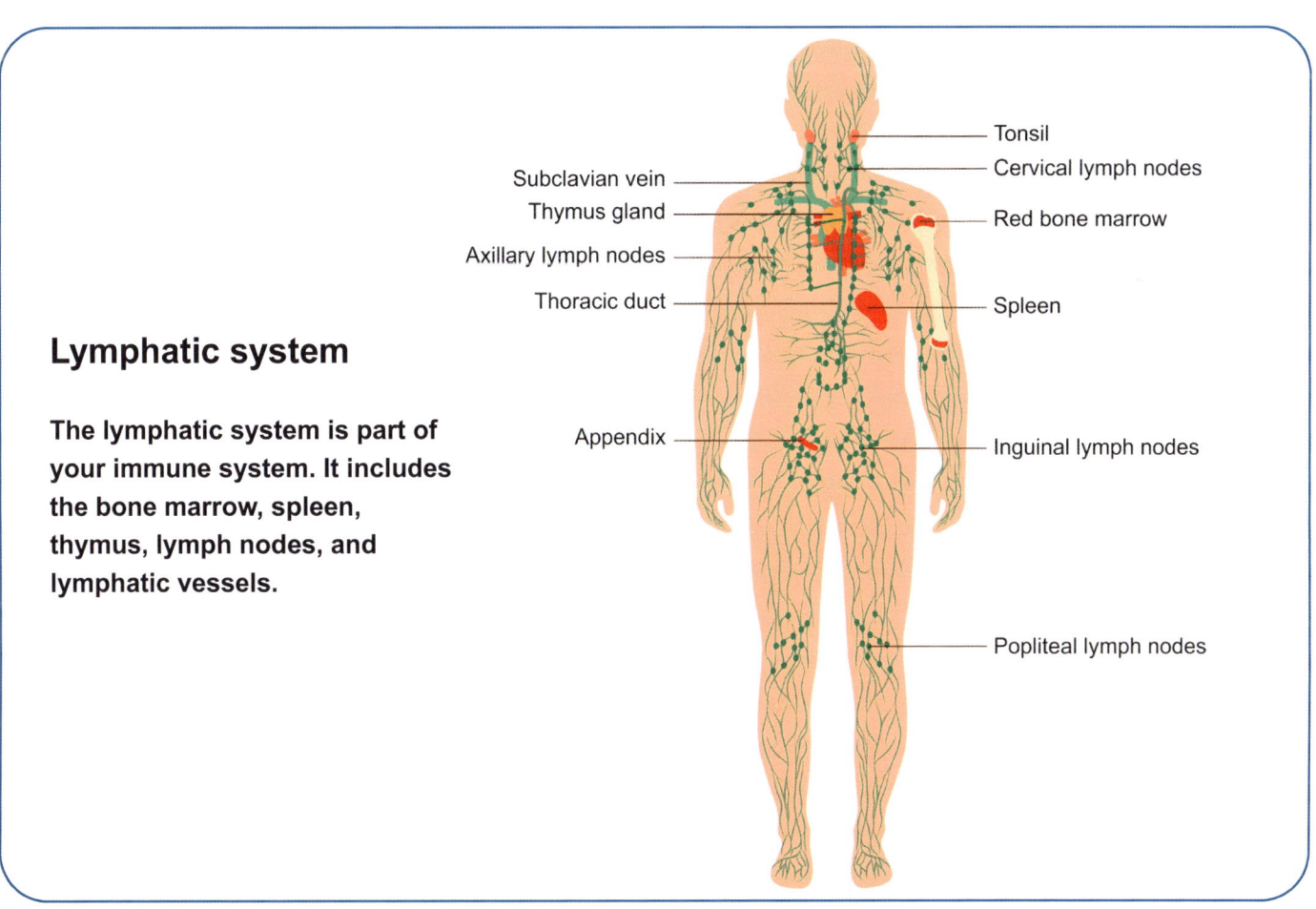

Lymphatic system

The lymphatic system is part of your immune system. It includes the bone marrow, spleen, thymus, lymph nodes, and lymphatic vessels.

NCCN Guidelines for Patients®
Mycosis Fungoides/Sézary Syndrome, 2021

1 MF/SS basics | Lymphocytes

Lymphocytes

A lymphocyte is a type of white blood cell. White blood cells fight infections. Lymphocytes are found in both blood and lymph tissue. Lymph tissue includes lymph vessels and lymph nodes.

There are 3 main types of lymphocytes:

- B lymphocytes or B cells make antibodies. An antibody is a protein.
- T lymphocytes or T cells help kill tumor cells and help control immune responses.
- Natural killer (NK) cells have granules (small particles) with enzymes that can kill tumor cells or cells infected with a virus.

Lymphocytes normally grow in response to infection or inflammation. When they grow on their own, they can develop into a lymphoma.

T cell

T lymphocytes or T cells are direct fighters of foreign invaders and also produce cytokines, which help activate other parts of the immune system. T cells destroy the body's own cells that have been taken over by viruses or that have become cancerous. You have normal T cells throughout your body, including in your skin.

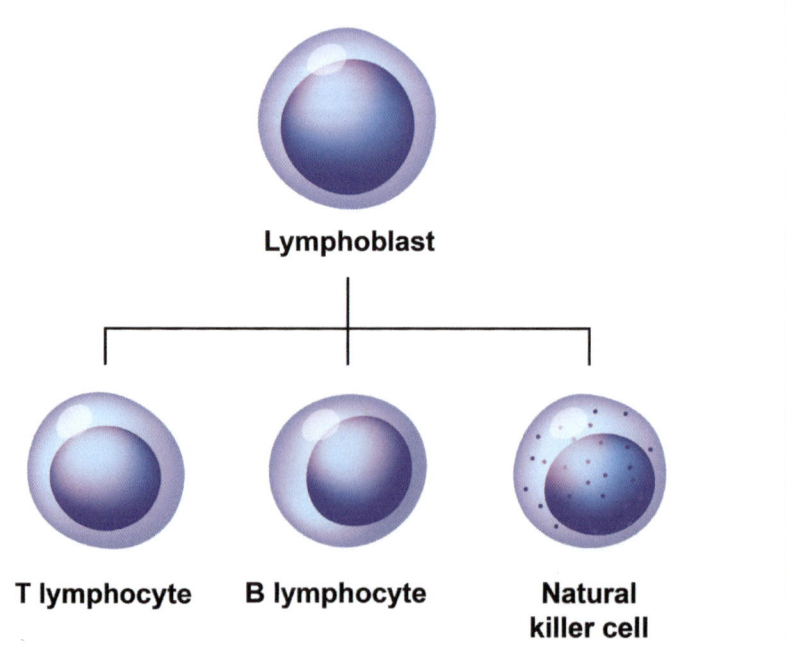

Lymphocytes

A lymphocyte is a type of white blood cell. In mycosis fungoides and Sézary syndrome abnormal T lymphocytes (T cells) cause skin lesions.

Cutaneous T-cell lymphoma

Cutaneous T-cell lymphoma (CTCL) is a rare form of non-Hodgkin lymphoma (NHL) that develops when abnormal T cells grow in the skin. These abnormal cells can grow in the blood, lymph nodes, or other areas of the body, as well. Although the skin is involved, the skin cells themselves are not cancerous.

On the skin, CTCL can cause rash-like redness, slightly raised or scaly, round patches, plaques, and sometimes skin tumors. The lesions are often itchy. Lesions may appear red, purple, or brown, and can be lighter in color than the surrounding skin. It might show up as more than one type of lesion and on different parts of the skin (often in areas not exposed to the sun). Some skin lymphomas appear as a red rash over some or most of the body (known as erythroderma).

CTCL is treatable, but generally not curable. You can live a long healthy life with ongoing care and management.

Types of CTCL include:

> Mycosis fungoides (MF) and Sézary syndrome (SS)
> Primary cutaneous CD30+ T-cell lymphoproliferative disorders

MF and SS are the most common forms of CTCL.

> In mycosis fungoides and Sézary syndrome, abnormal T lymphocytes can cause rashes, skin lesions, lymph node involvement, or abnormal blood counts.

About this book
This book will discuss treatment options for MF and SS.

More information on other types of CTCLs, primary cutaneous B-cell lymphomas (CBCLs), and primary cutaneous lymphomas (PCLs) can be found at NCCN.org/patientguidelines.

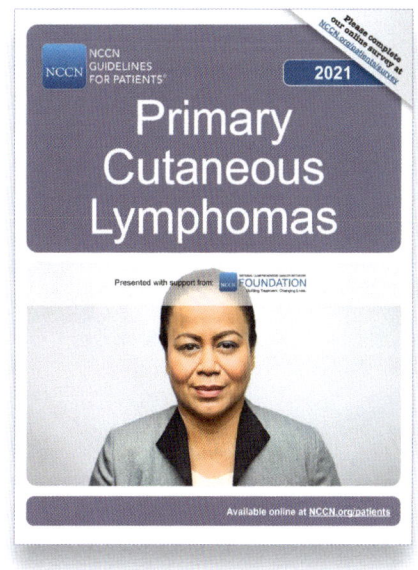

Mycosis fungoides

Mycosis fungoides (MF) is the most common form of cutaneous T-cell lymphoma (CTCL). It starts in the skin, but in those with more advanced skin involvement, MF can spread to the lymph nodes, blood, or other organs such as the spleen, liver, or lungs. Although the skin is involved, the skin cells themselves are not cancerous.

MF is usually indolent (slow-growing) and appears as patches, plaques, and tumors. A combination of patches, plaques, and tumors with open sores (ulceration) is possible. Symptoms include rash, tumors, skin lesions, and itchy skin.

There are several different types of MF:

- Folliculotropic mycosis fungoides (FMF) affects hair follicles, but not the uppermost layer of the skin (epidermis). Lesions are found in the head, eyebrow, or neck area and often with follicular papules and plaques. Loss of hair is common in affected sites.

- Pagetoid reticulosis (PR) or Woringer-Kolopp disease is characterized mostly by a single, persistent, scaly plaque, commonly involving the limbs.

- Granulomatous slack skin (GSS) is extremely rare and appears as bulky, hanging skin folds in the armpit or groin.

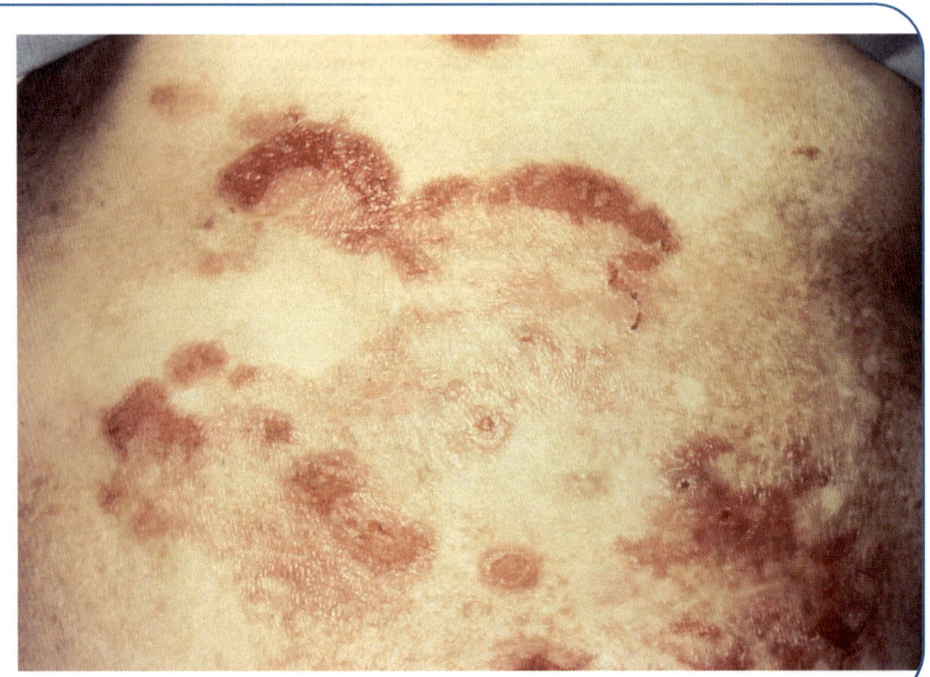

Mycosis fungoides

An example of mycosis fungoides skin lesions.

Credit: CDC/ Richard S. Hibbits. https://phil.cdc.gov/Details.aspx?pid=15467

1 MF/SS basics — Sézary syndrome

Sézary syndrome

Sézary syndrome (SS) is a rare type of cutaneous T-cell lymphoma (CTCL) that presents with blood involvement and often causes skin redness over most of the body (erythroderma). In SS, abnormal T cells called Sézary cells are found in the skin and blood, and may cause swollen and enlarged lymph nodes (lymphadenopathy). A characteristic of Sézary cells is an abnormally shaped nucleus, described as cerebriform.

> In Sézary syndrome, cancerous T cells called Sézary cells are found in the skin, lymph nodes, and blood.

Sézary syndrome

A characteristic of Sézary cells is an abnormally shaped nucleus, described as cerebriform.

Credit: https://commons.wikimedia.org/wiki/File:Hem1SezaryCell.jpg

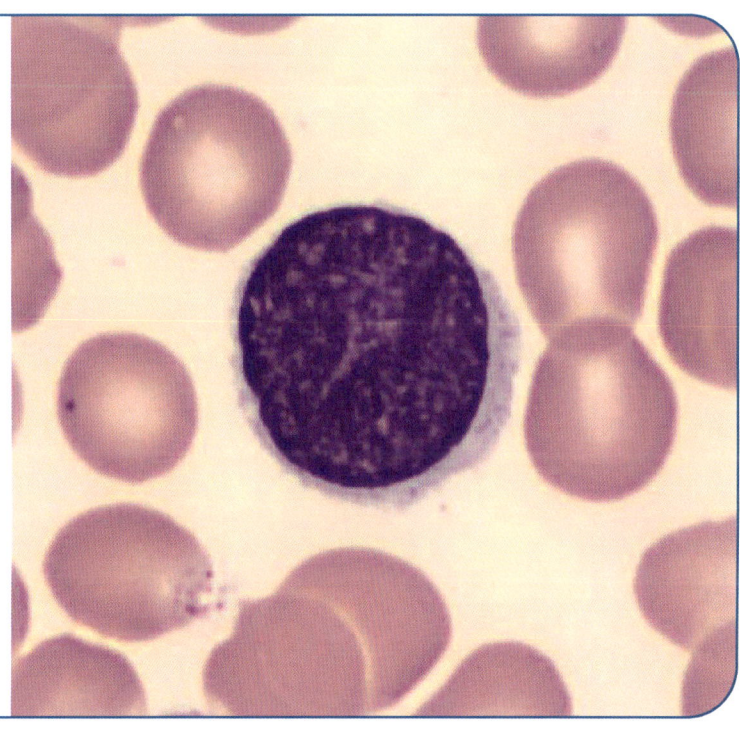

1 MF/SS basics | Review

Review

- The lymphatic or lymph system is a network of tissues and organs that helps your body fight infections and disease. It is part of the immune system.

- Lymphoma is a broad term for cancer that begins in a type of white blood cell called a lymphocyte. Lymphocytes fight infections.

- Primary cutaneous lymphomas (PCLs) are a rare group of non-Hodgkin lymphomas that cause skin lesions that are different from skin cancer.

- Cutaneous T-cell lymphoma (CTCL) is a rare form of cancer that develops when T lymphocytes grow and multiply uncontrollably in the skin.

- Mycosis fungoides (MF) is the most common form of CTCL.

- In Sézary syndrome (SS), cancerous T cells called Sézary cells are found in the skin, blood, and lymph nodes.

> Those with primary cutaneous T-cell lymphoma should be treated at centers experienced in this type of cancer.

2
Testing for MF/SS

14	Test results	25	Cancer stages
15	General health tests	29	Review
17	Skin exam		
19	Blood tests		
20	Imaging tests		
21	Biopsy		
23	Tissue tests		
24	Molecular tests		

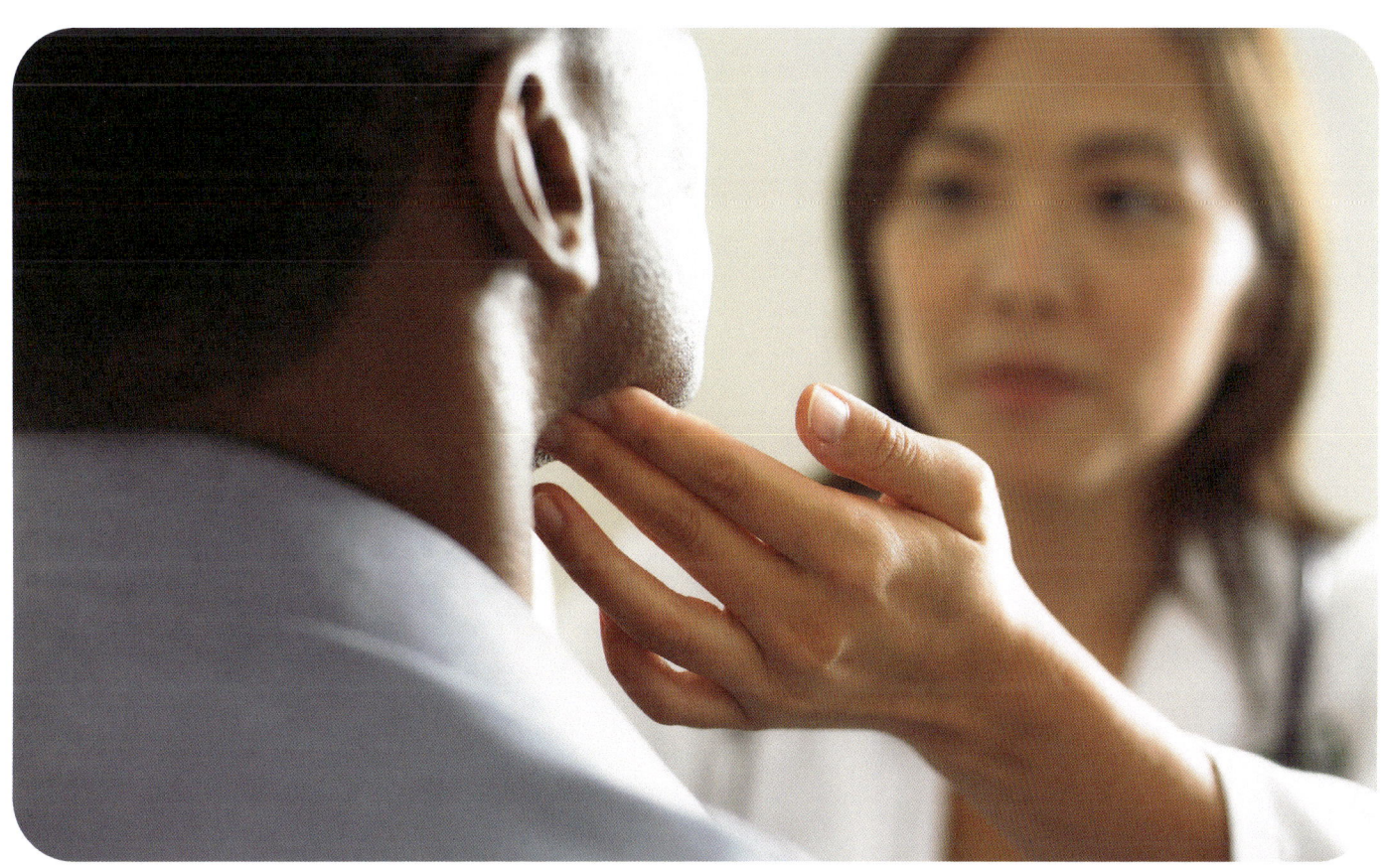

2 Testing for MF/SS | Test results

Treatment planning starts with testing. Accurate testing is needed to diagnose and treat MF/SS. This chapter presents an overview of the tests you might receive and what to expect.

Test results

The diagnosis of mycosis fungoides (MF) and Sézary syndrome (SS) is based primarily on a skin biopsy. Examination of the blood can detect circulating cancer cells and is part of diagnosing SS. Results of your physical exam, blood tests, skin biopsy, and possible imaging studies will determine your treatment plan. It is important you understand what these tests mean.

Keep these things in mind:

- Bring someone with you to doctor visits, if possible.
- Write down questions and take notes during appointments. Don't be afraid to ask your care team questions. Get to know your care team and let them get to know you.
- Get copies of blood tests, imaging results, and reports about the specific type of cancer you have.
- Organize your papers. Create files for insurance forms, medical records, and test results. You can do the same on your computer.
- Keep a list of contact information for everyone on your care team. Add it to your phone. Hang the list on your fridge or keep it in a place where someone can access it in an emergency.

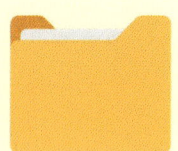

Create a medical binder

A medical binder or notebook is a great way to organize all of your records in one place.

- Make copies of blood tests, imaging results, and reports about your specific type of cancer. It will be helpful when getting a second opinion.
- Choose a binder that meets your needs. Consider a zipper pocket to include a pen, small calendar, and insurance cards.
- Create folders for insurance forms, medical records, and tests results. You can do the same on your computer.
- Use online patient portals to view your test results and other records. Download or print the records to add to your binder.
- Organize your binder in a way that works for you. Add a section for questions and to take notes.
- Bring your medical binder to appointments. You never know when you might need it!

2 Testing for MF/SS | General health tests

General health tests

Medical history
A medical history is a record of all health issues and treatments you have had in your life. Be prepared to list any illness or injury and when it happened. Bring a list of old and new medicines and any over-the-counter medicines, herbals, or supplements you take. Tell your doctor about any symptoms you have. A medical history will help determine which treatment is best for you.

Family history
Some cancers and other diseases can run in families. Your doctor will ask about the health history of family members who are blood relatives. This information is called a family history. Ask family members about their health issues like heart disease, cancer, and diabetes, and at what age they were diagnosed.

Physical exam
During a physical exam, a health care provider may:

- Check your temperature, blood pressure, pulse, and breathing rate
- Weigh you
- Listen to your lungs and heart
- Look in your eyes, ears, nose, and throat
- Feel and apply pressure to parts of your body to see if organs are of normal size, are soft or hard, or cause pain when touched.
- Feel for enlarged lymph nodes in your neck, underarm, and groin.
- Conduct a complete skin exam.

Doctors should perform a thorough physical exam, including skim exam, with a complete health history.

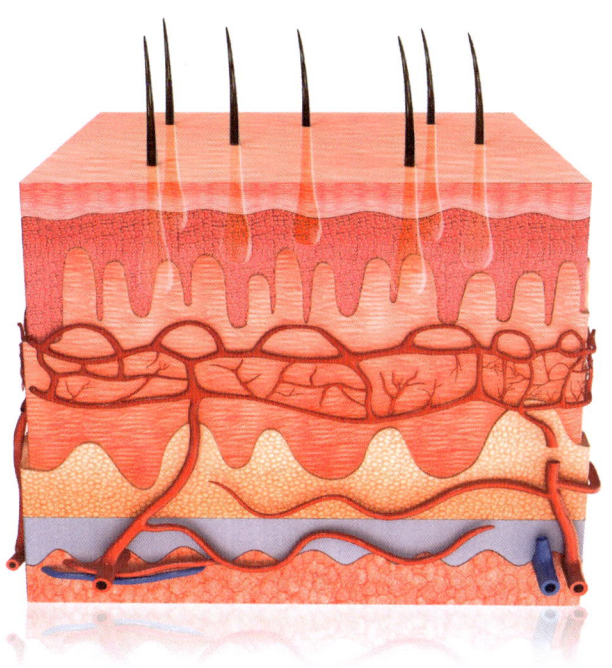

The skin

Mycosis fungoides and Sézary syndrome develop in the skin and can look like a rash, bumps, lumps, or tumor.

| 2 | Testing for MF/SS | | General health tests |

For possible tests, see Guide 1.

Ask questions and keep copies of your test results. Online patient portals are a great way to access your test results.

Guide 1 Testing

Needed	Medical history
	Physical exam that includes applying pressure to lymph nodes and internal organs
	Complete skin exam identifying body surface area (BSA) and type of lesion
	Complete blood count (CBC) with differential and absolute lymphocyte count
	Sézary count in blood by performing flow cytometry
	Tests to detect clonal T-cell antigen receptor (*TCR*) gene rearrangement in peripheral blood lymphocytes if blood involvement suspected
	Comprehensive metabolic panel (CMP) and lactate dehydrogenase (LDH)
	Chest, abdomen, pelvis CT with contrast or whole body PET/CT (arms/legs included of entire body when needed) (these may not be done in early-stage disease)
In some cases	Bone marrow biopsy in those with unexplained abnormal blood cell counts
	Biopsy of enlarged lymph nodes or suspected sites other than skin (if biopsy of skin is not diagnostic). Rebiopsy may be needed.
	Rebiopsy skin if suspicious of large-cell transformed (LCT) or folliculotropic MF
	Whole body PET/CT scan. A CT scan of neck, chest, abdomen, pelvis with contrast may also be requested
	Pregnancy test if treatment might affect pregnancy
	Discussion of fertility and sperm banking, if treatment might affect fertility

2 Testing for MF/SS — Skin exam

Skin exam

It is important to find an experienced dermatologist to conduct a skin exam. A complete skin exam looks for signs of MF/SS. MF/SS might appear as a rash, lumps, bumps, or tumor. A rash is an area of irritated or swollen skin. Many rashes are itchy, red, painful, and irritated. As a rash, MF/SS might come and go.

MF/SS is a chronic disease that can come and go with or without treatment. Keeping a photo journal might help track your skin changes over time.

The amount of cancer is measured using the size of your hand. One hand is equal to 1 percent (1%) of your total body surface area (BSA). In addition, any tumors will be measured by their depth, height, size, and region of the body.

The skin

Skin is the largest organ in your body. Not only does it protect your body, but it tells doctors a lot about your health. Doctors take your pulse and blood pressure through your skin. They notice if the skin feels warm, hot, or cool to the touch.

A skin lesion is a change in skin color or texture. Skin lesions can appear anywhere on the body, but are most common on the lower abdomen, upper thighs, buttocks, and breasts. Some words to describe skin lesions might include patch, papule, plaque, nodule, tumor, and erythroderma.

Skin lesions

A papule is a very small, solid bump. A plaque is a raised or hardened lesion that forms on the skin, larger than a papule. Plaques sometimes become tumors on the skin.

Credit: https://commons.wikimedia.org/wiki/File:Papule_and_Plaque.svg

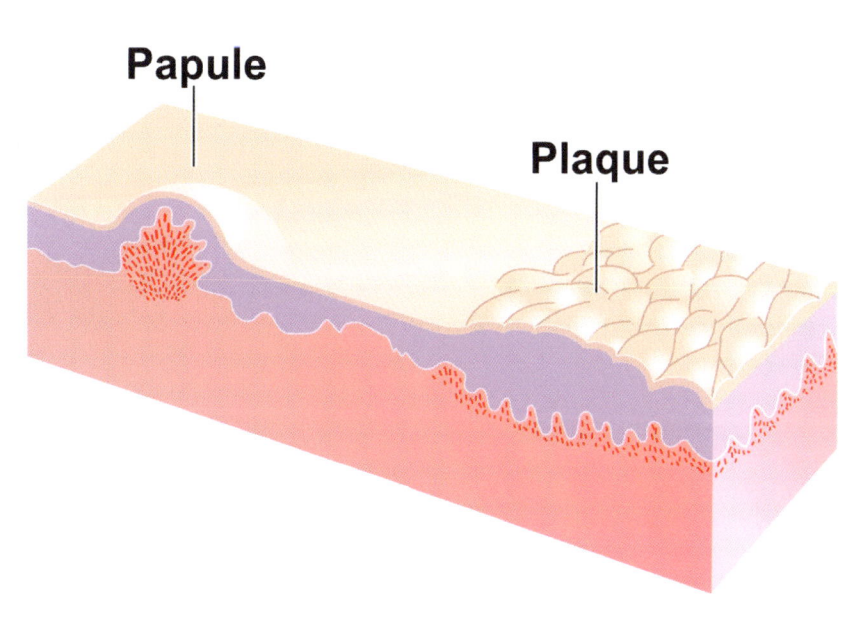

Patch
A patch is a flat, thin, pink or red lesion of any size that forms on the skin. Patches may be dry, scaly, and itchy, and may look like eczema or psoriasis. They can be lighter than surrounding skin or brown in people with darker skin. The patches may sometimes become plaques (hard, raised lesions) on the skin.

Papule
A papule is a very small, solid lump that might look like a very small pimple. Papules may be red, purple, brown, or pink. Papules can be found in groups.

Plaque
A plaque is a raised (elevated) or hardened (indurated) lesion of any size that forms on the skin. Plaques may be red, scaly, and itchy and may look like eczema or psoriasis. Plaques sometimes become tumors on the skin.

Erythroderma
Erythroderma is redness of over 80% of the body's skin surface. It is an important part of recognizing and treating MF/SS. Erythroderma can look like a sunburn or large blotches on the skin.

Tumor
A tumor is a firm, dome-shaped mass at least 1 centimeter in size.

Ulcer
A skin ulcer is an open sore or wound on the skin caused by poor blood flow.

> Keeping a photo journal might help track your skin changes over time.

Skin color
Melanin gives your skin color. Skin color is based on the amount of melanin in your skin, and the amount of oxygen and hemoglobin in your blood. Hemoglobin is a protein found inside red blood cells. Testing for the amount of hemoglobin in the blood is usually part of a complete blood count (CBC) test.

You know your skin better than anyone. Tell your doctor about your normal skin color. Show your doctor the differences in where the skin looks normal and different to you. Describe any changes. Does the area itch or burn? Is it dry? Is it red or warm to the touch? Are there bumps or a raised smooth area? Is there an odor? Share any photos.

Blood tests

Blood tests check for signs of disease and how well organs are working. They require a sample of your blood, which is removed through a needle placed into your vein.

Complete blood count
A complete blood count (CBC) measures the levels of red blood cells (RBCs), white blood cells (WBCs), and platelets in your blood. Your doctor will want to know if you have enough red blood cells to carry oxygen throughout your body, white blood cells to fight infection, and platelets to control bleeding.

Comprehensive metabolic panel
A comprehensive metabolic panel (CMP) measures 14 different substances in your blood. It is usually done on the plasma part of your blood. A CMP provides important information about how well your kidneys and liver are working, among other things.

Differential
There are 5 types of white blood cells: neutrophils, lymphocytes, monocytes, eosinophils, and basophils. A differential counts the number of each type of WBC. It also checks if the counts are in balance with each other.

HTLV
Human T-lymphotropic virus (HTLV) testing is used to detect an infection by HTLV-I or HTLV-II. A blood test is used to detect an HTLV infection that could be the cause of a T-cell lymphoma. In the United States, all donated blood is screened for HTLV.

Lactic acid
Lactate dehydrogenase (LDH) or lactic acid dehydrogenase is an enzyme found in most cells. Dying cells release LDH into blood. Fast-growing cells, such as tumor cells, also release LDH.

Pregnancy test
If planned treatment might affect pregnancy, then those who can become pregnant will be given a pregnancy test before treatment begins.

Imaging tests

Imaging tests take pictures (images) of the inside of your body. These tests are used to look for cancer in organs and areas outside of the blood. A radiologist, an expert in test images, will write a report and send this report to your doctor. Your doctor will discuss the results with you.

CT scan

A computed tomography (CT or CAT) scan uses x-rays and computer technology to take pictures of the inside of the body. It takes many x-rays of the same body part from different angles. All the images are combined to make one detailed picture. In most cases, contrast will be used. Contrast materials are not dyes, but substances that help certain areas in the body stand out. They are used to make the pictures clearer. Contrast materials are not permanent and will leave the body in your urine.

Tell your doctors if you have had bad reactions to contrast in the past. This is important. You might be given medicines, such as Benadryl® and prednisone, for an allergy to contrast. Contrast might not be used if you have a serious allergy or if your kidneys aren't working well.

MRI scan

A magnetic resonance imaging (MRI) scan uses radio waves and powerful magnets to take pictures of the inside of the body. It does not use x-rays. Contrast might be used.

PET scan

A positron emission tomography (PET) scan uses a radioactive drug called a tracer. A tracer is a substance injected into a vein to see where it is in the body and if it is using sugar to grow. Cancer cells show up as bright spots on PET scans. Not all bright spots are cancer. It is normal for the brain, heart, kidneys, and bladder to be bright on PET. When a PET scan is combined with CT, it is called a PET/CT scan.

2 Testing for MF/SS | Biopsy

Biopsy

A biopsy is the removal of a sample tissue or a group of cells for testing. A biopsy is needed to diagnose mycosis fungoides (MF) and Sézary syndrome (SS). Your sample should be reviewed by a pathologist who is an expert in the diagnosis of MF/SS. The pathologist will review thin sections of the skin biopsy under a microscope. This review is often referred to as histology or histopathology review. The pathologist will note the overall appearance and the size, shape, and type of your cells.

Histology is the study of the anatomy (structure) of cells, tissues, and organs under a microscope. Follicular mycosis fungoides (FMF) and large-cell transformation (LCT) are two histology features that can be found in any disease stage.

A biopsy is an important part of a correct MF/SS diagnosis. See Guide 2.

Guide 2
Diagnosis

Needed	Biopsy of suspicious skin sites (multiple biopsies may be needed)
	Biopsy review done by pathologist who is an expert in the diagnosis of cutaneous T-cell lymphomas (CTCLs)
	Immunohistochemistry (IHC) panel of skin biopsy to include: • CD2, CD3, CD4, CD5, CD7, CD8, CD20, CD30
	Molecular analysis or other test to detect clonal T-cell antigen receptor (*TCR*) gene rearrangements
In some cases	Blood test to look for Sézary cells
	IHC panel of skin biopsy to include: • CD25, CD56, TIA1, granzyme B, TCRß, TCRδ, CXCL13, ICOS, and PD-1
	Biopsy of enlarged lymph nodes or suspected sites other than skin (if biopsy of skin is not diagnostic)
	Assessment of HTLV-1/2

Skin lesion biopsy

A sample of your lesion will be removed and tested to confirm MF/SS. A skin lesion biopsy can be incisional or excisional. An incisional biopsy removes an area of skin using a scalpel blade. Stitches are usually required after an incisional biopsy. An excisional biopsy usually removes a larger area of skin and is done infrequently in MF/SS.

Diagnosing MF/SS can be a challenge. It is common to have several skin biopsies in order to make a clear diagnosis.

Skin punch biopsy

In a skin punch biopsy, a small piece of skin and connective tissue are removed using a hand-held tool. Stitches are often used to close the opening in the skin.

Skin shave biopsy

A skin shave biopsy removes a shaving of the top layer of skin using a tool similar to a razor. This type of biopsy is not recommended for very flat skin lesions because it doesn't take a deep enough sample. Abnormal T cells are often found under the surface of the skin.

Lymph node biopsy

A lymph node might be biopsied if cancer is suspected based on a test or physical exam. Lymph nodes are usually too small to be seen or felt. Sometimes, lymph nodes can feel swollen, enlarged, hard to the touch, or don't move when pushed (fixed or immobile). This is called palpable adenopathy or lymphadenopathy. A lymph node biopsy can be done using a needle biopsy procedure or as a small surgery to remove a lymph node.

Bone marrow tests

Bone marrow tests are very rare in MF/SS and might be done in those with unexplained abnormal blood cells.

There are 2 types of bone marrow tests that are often done at the same time:

- Bone marrow aspirate
- Bone marrow biopsy

Your bone marrow is like a sponge holding liquid and cells. An aspirate takes some of the liquid and cells out of the sponge, and a biopsy takes a piece of the sponge.

The samples are usually taken from the back of the hip bone (pelvis). You will likely lie on your belly or side. Your doctors will first clean and give sedation or numb your skin and outer surface of your bone. For an aspirate, a hollow needle will be pushed through your skin and into the bone. Liquid bone marrow will then be drawn into a syringe. For the biopsy, a wider needle will be used to remove a core sample. You may feel bone pain at your hip for a few days. Your skin may bruise.

2 Testing for MF/SS | Tissue tests

Tissue tests

Tissue and cells removed during a skin biopsy will be tested.

Immunophenotyping

Immunophenotyping is a process that uses antibodies to detect the presence or absence of T-cell antigens. Antigens are proteins or markers that can be found on the surface of or inside white blood cells such as T cells. Specific groupings of antigens are normal. However, some specific patterns of antigens are found on abnormal cells.

Immunophenotyping can be done using flow cytometry or immunohistochemistry (IHC). Flow cytometry immunophenotyping in blood may be used to help diagnose and treat MF/SS. MF and SS cells are typically characterized by the following immunophenotype: CD2+, CD3+, CD5+, CD4+, CD8- (rarely CD8+), and they lack certain T-cell markers, such as CD7- and CD26-. Immunophenotype can change as cancer progresses.

Flow cytometry

Flow cytometry is a laboratory method used to detect, identify, and count specific cells. Flow cytometry involves adding a light-sensitive dye to cells. The dyed cells are passed through a beam of light in a machine. The machine measures the number of cells, things like the size and shape of the cells, and proteins on the surface of thousands of cells. Flow cytometry may be used on cells from circulating (peripheral) blood, lymph nodes, skin, or tumors. The most common use of flow cytometry is in the identification of markers on cells, particularly in the immune system (called immunophenotyping).

Immunohistochemistry

Immunohistochemistry (IHC) is a special staining process that involves adding a chemical marker to detect immune cells on histology studies to see which proteins they express. The cells are then studied using a microscope. IHC looks for the immunophenotype of cells from a skin biopsy.

CD4 and CD8 are proteins that are on two families of T lymphocytes. CD4 T cells (helper cells) help regulate functions of the immune system. CD8 T cells (killer cells) break down or rid the body of foreign substances. Most cases of CTCL come from CD4 T cells. An IHC will look for these cells and others. An IHC panel of skin biopsy may include testing for CD2, CD3, CD4, CD5, CD7, CD8, CD20, and CD30. Others might be included.

2 Testing for MF/SS | Molecular tests

Molecular tests

Molecular tests are used to learn more about your type of MF/SS and to target treatment. Talk to your care team and/or a genetic counselor about your family history of cancer.

Inside our cells are deoxyribonucleic acid (DNA) molecules. These molecules are tightly packaged into what is called a chromosome. Chromosomes contain most of the genetic information in a cell. Normal human cells contain 23 pairs of chromosomes for a total of 46 chromosomes. Each chromosome contains thousands of genes. Genes tell cells what to do and what to become.

Molecular or biomarker testing looks for specific proteins or molecules. Genes are written like this: *TCR*. Proteins are written like this: CD4.

Comparative genomic hybridization
Comparative genomic hybridization (CGH) is a technique that compares DNA samples from normal tissue and tumor tissue. It is used to detect abnormal chromosomes.

High-throughput sequencing
High-throughput sequencing (HTS) is capable of sequencing hundreds of millions of DNA molecules at a time.

Next-generation sequencing
Next-generation sequencing (NGS) is a high-throughput method used to determine a portion of a person's DNA sequence.

PCR
A polymerase chain reaction (PCR) is a lab process that can make millions or billions of copies of your DNA (genetic information) in just a few hours, but results can take days. PCR is very sensitive. It can find 1 abnormal cell among more than 100,000 normal cells.

T-cell antigen receptor
When one T cell divides many times to form a tumor, the entire group of cells is called clonal. Each T cell has a unique T-cell receptor. If there is clonal proliferation of T cells as can be seen in MF/SS, then all cells of the tumor have the same T-cell antigen receptor. Molecular testing (analysis) is used to detect clonal T-cell antigen receptor (*TCR*) gene rearrangements. This information is helpful when diagnosing MF/SS.

| 2 | Testing for MF/SS | Cancer stages |

Cancer stages

A cancer stage is a way to describe the extent of the cancer at the time you are first diagnosed. The American Joint Committee on Cancer (AJCC) created this to determine how much cancer is in your body, where it is located, and what subtype you have. This is called staging. Staging is needed to make treatment decisions.

For MF/SS staging, see Guide 3.

Guide 3
MF/SS cancer stages

Stage 1	**Stage 1A** (Limited skin involvement)	• T1, N0, M0, B0 or B1
	Stage 1B (Skin only disease)	• T2, N0, M0, B0 or B1
Stage 2	**Stage 2A**	• T1 or T2, N1 or N2, M0, B0 or B1
	Stage 2B (Tumor stage disease)	• T3, N0 or N1 or N2, M0, B0 or B1
Stage 3	**Stage 3A** (Erythrodermic disease)	• T4, N0 or N1 or N2, M0, B0
	Stage 3B (Erythrodermic disease)	• T4, N0 or N1 or N2, M0, B1
Stage 4	**Stage 4A$_1$** (Sézary syndrome)	• Any T, N0 or N1 or N2, M0, B2
	Stage 4A$_2$ (Sézary syndrome or non-Sézary)	• Any T, N3, M0, Any B
	Stage 4B (Visceral disease)	• Any T, Any N, M1, Any B

NCCN Guidelines for Patients®
Mycosis Fungoides/Sézary Syndrome, 2021

2 Testing for MF/SS | Cancer stages

TNMB scores

The tumor, node, metastasis (TNM) system is used to stage many cancers. In this system, the letters T, N, and M describe different areas of cancer growth. Based on biopsy and other test results, your doctor will assign a score or number to each letter. The higher the number, the larger the tumor or the more the cancer has spread to lymph nodes or other organs. These scores will be combined to assign the cancer a stage. A TNM example might look like this: T1N0M0 or T1, N0, M0.

Staging in MF/SS looks slightly different than other cancers. It is referred to as TNMB or tumor, node, metastasis, blood.

- **T is for skin** – In MF/SS, tumor refers to type and number of tumors covering the skin. Staging looks for the presence of tumors, patches, papules, plaques, or reddening of the skin (erythema) and how much body surface area (BSA) is affected.

- **N is for node** – This refers to if abnormal T lymphocytes are found in lymph nodes.

- **M is for visceral** - In MF/SS, visceral refers to if cancer is found in internal organs.

- **B is for blood** – If abnormal T lymphocytes are found in circulating (peripheral) blood.

Numbered stages

Number stages range from stage 1 to stage 4, with 4 being the most advanced. These stages are written as stage I, stage II, stage III, and stage IV. Not all cancers are described this way. Stages are defined by TNMB scores.

T = Skin

In MF/SS, the amount of cancer is measured by evaluating what percent of your skin is affected by lymphoma. One hand is equal to 1 percent (1%) of your total body surface area (BSA). In addition, any tumors will be measured by their depth, height, size, and region of the body. Tumors are often measured in centimeters (cm).

- **T1** – Patches, papules, and/or plaques cover less than 10% BSA

- **T2** – Patches, papules, and/or plaques cover 10% or more BSA
  - **T2a** is patch only
  - **T2b** is plaque with or without patch

- **T3** – One or more tumors of 1 cm or more in size

- **T4** – Reddening, thickening, or involvement of the skin (erythema) covering 80% or more BSA

N = Node

There are hundreds of lymph nodes throughout your body. Lymph nodes work as filters to help fight infection and remove harmful things. They also produce lymphocytes. As abnormal T lymphocytes multiply, they can distort or overtake the lymph node.

Abnormal lymph nodes are any that can be felt on physical exam as firm, irregular, clustered, fixed, or 1.5 cm or more in diameter. Node groups examined on physical exam include neck (cervical), above the collarbone (supraclavicular), arm (epitrochlear), armpit (axillary), and groin (inguinal).

- **N0** means no abnormal T lymphocytes are found
- **N1** means some abnormal T lymphocytes are found
- **N2** means many abnormal T lymphocytes or clusters are found
- **N3** means abnormal T lymphocytes have altered the structure of lymph node. This is called lymph node (nodal) disease and is stage 4.

M = Visceral

Cancer that has spread to distant parts of the body is usually called metastatic. It is shown as M1. In MF/SS cancer spreads to visceral (internal) organs such as the spleen, liver, or lungs.

- **M0** means no cancer is found in visceral organs
- **M1** means cancer is found in visceral organs

B = Blood

Peripheral blood circulates throughout your body (bloodstream). The amount of abnormal T cells found in the blood will be measured.

- **B0** (very low blood involvement) – No blood involvement or very small amounts (less than 15%, less than 250 cells/mm^3) of CD4+/CD26- or CD4+/CD7- cells or other abnormal T lymphocytes are found.
- **B1** (low blood tumor burden) – More than 5% of peripheral blood lymphocytes are Sézary cells. Or, more than 15% of total lymphocytes or more than 250 cells/mm^3 are CD4+/CD26- or CD4+/CD7-, or other abnormal T lymphocytes.
- **B2** (high blood tumor burden) – More than 1000/mcL Sézary cells are found. Or, CD4+/CD26- (more than 30% of lymphocytes), CD4+/CD7- (more than 40% of lymphocytes), or other abnormal T lymphocytes are found in both skin and blood. A diagnosis of Sézary syndrome requires B2 involvement.

Stage 1A – Limited skin involvement
Limited patches, papules, and/or plaques cover less than 10% of the skin (T1). Cancer is not found in lymph nodes (N0) or visceral organs (M0). If cancer is found in the blood (B1), it might be treated as stage 3 erythrodermic disease.

Stage 1B – Skin only disease
Stage 1B has more extensive skin involvement than stage 1A, but no disease outside the skin. Patches, papules, and/or plaques cover 10% or more of the skin (T2). Cancer is not found in lymph nodes (N0) or visceral organs (M0). If cancer is found in the blood (B1), it might be treated as stage 3 erythrodermic disease.

Stage 2A
Any amount of the skin surface is covered with patches or plaques (T1 or T2). Cancer is found in the lymph nodes (N1 or N2). If cancer is found in the blood (B1), it might be treated as stage 3 erythrodermic disease.

Stage 2B – Tumor stage disease
One or more tumors 1 cm or more in size are found on the skin (T3). Cancer may (N1 or N2) or may not (N0) be in the lymph nodes. It may or may not be found in blood (B1 or B0).

Stage 3A – Erythrodermic disease
In erythrodermic disease, nearly all of the skin is reddened (erythema) (T4), but no significant disease outside the skin. Patches, plaques, or tumors may be present. Cancer may (N1 or N2) or may not (N0) be in the lymph nodes. There is no visceral (M0) or blood (B0) involvement.

Stage 3B – Erythrodermic disease
In erythrodermic disease, nearly all of the skin is reddened (erythema) (T4) and there are some signs of disease outside the skin (in the blood or lymph nodes). Patches, plaques, or tumors may be present. Cancer may (N1 or N2) or may not (N0) be in the lymph nodes. There is no visceral (M0) involvement. Cancer is found in blood (B1).

Stage $4A_1$ – Sézary syndrome
Stage $4A_1$ has more significant disease in the blood. When there is a high number of Sézary cells in the blood, it is called Sézary syndrome. Skin can be any stage (any T). Cancer may (N1 or N2) or may not (N0) be in the lymph nodes. A high number of Sézary cells are found in blood (B2).

Stage $4A_2$ – Sézary syndrome or non-Sézary
Stage $4A_2$ has more significant disease in the lymph nodes. Skin can be any stage (any T). Abnormal T lymphocytes have altered the structure of the lymph node (N3). Cancer may be found in blood. A diagnosis of Sézary syndrome requires B2 involvement.

Stage 4B – Visceral disease
Stage 4B has more significant disease in the organs. Skin can be any stage (any T). Lymph nodes can be any stage (any N). Cancer has spread to internal (visceral) organs (M1). There may be blood involvement (any B).

2 Testing for MF/SS | Review

Review

- Tests are used to plan treatment and check how well treatment is working.

- Online portals are a great way to access your test results.

- Skin lesions can appear anywhere on the body, but are most common on the lower abdomen, upper thighs, buttocks, and breasts. Lesions may look like papules, patches, plaques, or tumors.

- Physical exam, blood, imaging, and tissue tests check for signs of disease.

- A biopsy is needed to diagnose mycosis fungoides (MF) and Sézary syndrome (SS). Your sample should be reviewed by a pathologist who is an expert in the diagnosis of MF/SS.

- A sample from your biopsy will be tested to look for biomarkers or proteins.

- A cancer stage is a way to describe the extent of the cancer at the time you are first diagnosed.

- The tumor, node, metastasis, blood (TNMB) system might be used to describe your cancer.

> Tell your doctor about any medicines, vitamins, over-the-counter drugs, herbals, or supplements you are taking.

3
Treating MF/SS

- 31 Overview
- 31 Multidisciplinary team
- 32 Pregnancy and fertility
- 32 Skin-directed therapy
- 34 Radiation therapy
- 35 Systemic therapy
- 36 Clinical trials
- 37 Stem cell transplant
- 38 Supportive care
- 39 Review

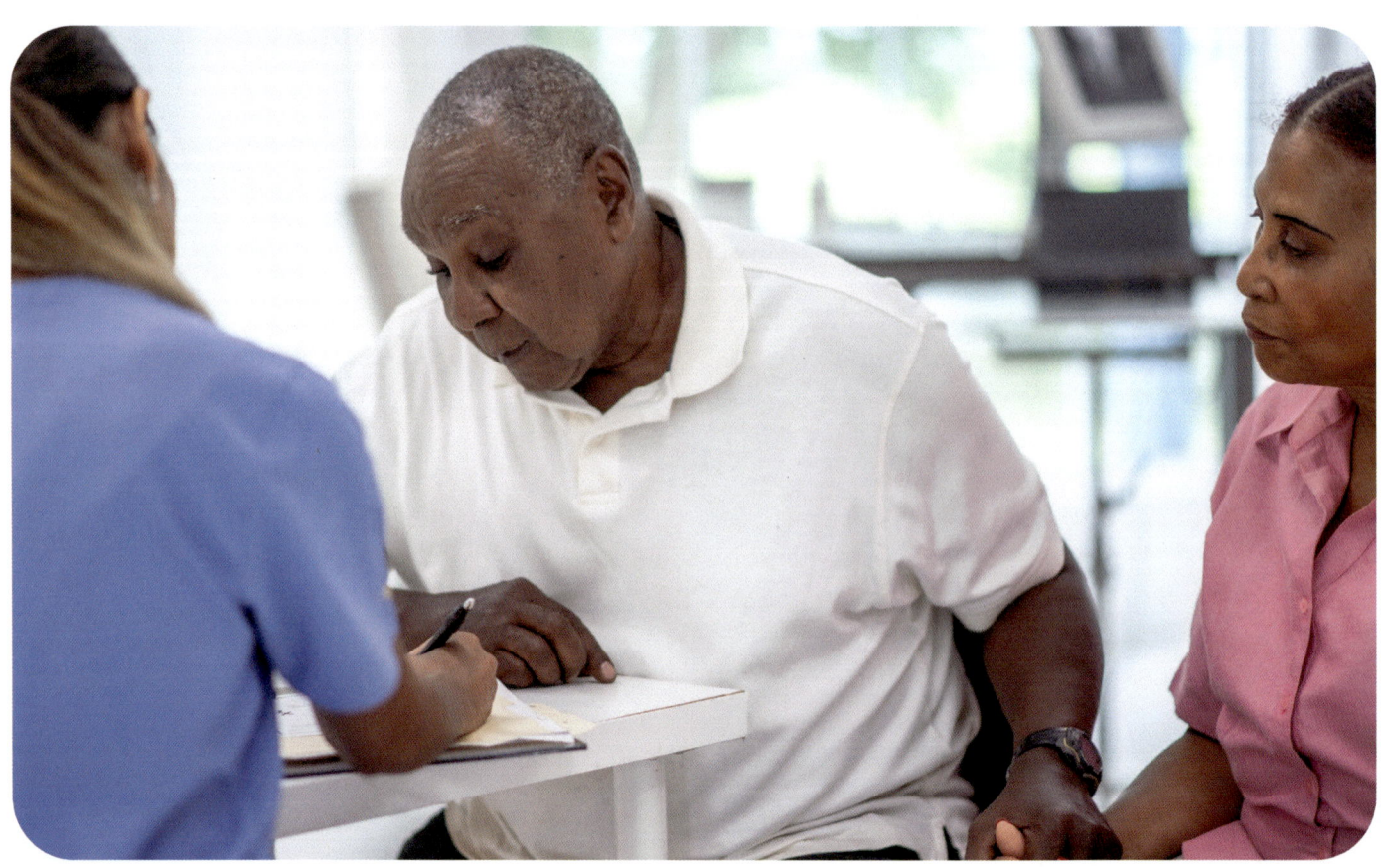

3 Treating MF/SS | Overview

This chapter is a general overview of the types of treatment for mycosis fungoides (MF) and Sézary syndrome (SS) and what to expect. Together, you and your doctor will chose a treatment plan that is right for you.

Overview

Treatment planning for MF/SS is based on the extent, severity, and type of skin disease. It is also based on if disease is found in the blood, lymph nodes, or other areas outside of the skin (extracutaneous). Your age, ability to perform daily tasks, if you have other serious health issues, and drug availability and affordability all play a role in treatment decisions. Your wishes are always important.

In early-stage disease (stage 1A to 2A), treatment focuses on skin-directed therapies. In advanced-stage disease (stage 2B to 4), systemic therapies may be given upfront, but often in combination with skin-directed therapies.

CTCL is treatable, but generally not curable unless one undergoes a stem cell transplant. You can live a long healthy life with ongoing care and management. Emphasis will be on supportive care. Supportive care is health care that relieves symptoms caused by MF/SS or its treatment and improves quality of life.

Multidisciplinary team

Those with mycosis fungoides (MF) and Sézary syndrome (SS) should seek treatment or consultation at centers with expertise in the management of MF/SS.

Treating MF/SS takes a team approach. Treatment decisions should involve a multidisciplinary team (MDT) or a team of doctors from different fields of medicine who have knowledge (expertise) and experience with your type of cancer. This is important. Ask who will coordinate your care.

The MDT should include the following:

- A dermatologist specializes in the diagnosis and treatment of skin diseases.
- A hematologist/oncologist specializes in blood diseases and cancers and their treatment.
- A pathologist interprets the cells and tissues removed during a biopsy or surgery and performs flow cytometry, immunohistochemistry, and genetic studies.
- A radiation oncologist prescribes and plans radiation therapy to treat cancer.
- A radiologist interprets the results of x-rays and other imaging tests.

Some members of your care team will be with you throughout cancer treatment, while others will only be there for parts of it. Get to know your care team and let them get to know you.

3 Treating MF/SS | Pregnancy and fertility

Keep a list of names and contact information for each member of your team. This will make it easier for you and anyone involved in your care to know whom to contact with questions or concerns.

You know your body better than anyone. Help other team members understand:

> How you feel
> What you need
> What is working and what is not
> Your goals for treatment

> Get to know your care team and let them get to know you.

Pregnancy and fertility

Some treatments used in advanced-stage disease might affect pregnancy and fertility in both sexes. Fertility is the ability to have children. If you think you want children in the future, ask your doctor how cancer and cancer treatment might change your fertility and sexual health. Also, birth control for both sexes might be recommended.

Skin-directed therapy

Types of therapy focused on the skin include topical therapy, local radiation, and phototherapy.

Topical therapy
Topical treatments are put on the surface of the skin. It might be a lotion, gel, or ointment. Types of topical therapy are described next.

Topical and intralesional corticosteroids
Steroid is the short name for corticosteroid. Steroids are man-made and are used to reduce inflammation. Steroids used to treat MF/SS can be topical or intralesional. An intralesional steroid is injected directly into a lesion on or immediately below the skin.

Steroids can cause short-term and long-term side effects. Ask your care team about possible side effects. Corticosteroids are not the same as the steroids used by some athletes.

3 Treating MF/SS — Skin-directed therapy

Topical nitrogen mustard
Nitrogen mustard (mechlorethamine hydrochloride) stops or slows the growth of cancer. It has been used since the 1950s to treat mycosis fungoides and other cutaneous T-cell lymphomas.

Topical retinoids
Retinoids are products related to vitamin A. Topical bexarotene (Targretin® gel) and topical tazarotene (Tazorac® Gel, Tazorac® Cream) are retinoids applied to the skin to treat lesions, patches, or plaques.

Topical carmustine
Carmustine is a chemotherapy that stops or slows the growth of cancer. Topical carmustine (BiCNU®) is applied to lesions.

Topical imiquimod
Topical imiquimod is used to treat certain types of flat, scaly growths on the skin. Brand names include Aldara® and Zyclara®.

Local radiation
Local radiation treats the skin lesion or tumor only. Involved-site radiation therapy (ISRT) is a type of local radiation. The type of radiation is usually electrons. Some patients may see a benefit with low doses of radiation.

Phototherapy
Phototherapy uses different ultraviolet (UV) light wavelengths to treat skin lesions or tumors.

Types include:

- Ultraviolet light B (UVB) – exposes the skin to an artificial UVB light source for a set length of time on a regular schedule.

- Narrowband ultraviolet light B (NB-UVB) – uses a very specific UV wavelength. This is why it is called narrowband.

- Photochemotherapy ultraviolet light A (PUVA) – combines psoralen (P) with UVA. Psoralen is a type of medicine taken by mouth (orally) that causes your skin to be sensitive to light. After taking psoralen, the skin is exposed to long-wave ultraviolet light.

- Ultraviolet light A1 (UVA1) - penetrates deep into the skin causing T cells to die.

Often, UVB or NB-UVB is used for patch or thin plaques and PUVA or UVA1 is used for thicker plaques or tumors.

UV can increase your risk of some skin cancers. Phototherapy may not be favored in those with a history of squamoproliferative skin neoplasms, basal cell carcinomas, or who have had melanoma.

Radiation therapy

Radiation therapy (RT) uses radiation from electrons, photons, x-rays, protons, gamma rays, and other sources to kill cancer cells and shrink tumors. RT can be given alone or with other treatments. Treatment may focus on individual plaques or tumors, a small area of the body, the entire surface of the skin, or specific lymph nodes. RT may be used as supportive care or palliative care to help ease pain or discomfort caused by cancer.

EBRT

External beam radiation therapy (EBRT) uses a machine outside of the body to aim radiation at the tumor(s) or areas of the body.

Common types of EBRT that may be used to treat your cancer include:

- Involved-site radiation therapy (ISRT) targets a specific area of skin. It can also be used to treat specific lymph nodes with cancer.

- Total skin electron beam therapy (TSEBT) treats the entire skin surface. You might stand on a rotating platform to receive this treatment.

Less common types of EBRT that may be used to treat your cancer include:

- Three-dimensional conformal radiation therapy (3D-CRT) uses computer software and CT images to aim beams that match the shape of the tumor.

- Intensity-modulated radiation therapy (IMRT) uses small beams of different strengths to match the shape of the tumor.

- Stereotactic body radiation therapy (SBRT) uses high-energy radiation beams to treat cancers in five or fewer treatments.

- Stereotactic radiosurgery (SRS) uses special equipment to position the body and give one precise, large dose of radiation.

- Particle beam RT uses protons, carbon ions, or other heavy ions to treat cancer.

Systemic therapy

Systemic therapy works throughout the body. It includes retinoids, chemotherapy, targeted therapy, and immunotherapy. Systemic therapy might be used alone or with other therapies.

Extracorporeal photopheresis
Photopheresis, also known as extracorporeal photopheresis (ECP), is a medical treatment that removes blood from the body using a machine. The machine separates out the white blood cells. These white cells are exposed to a medicine called 8-methoxypsoralen (8-MOP) followed by ultraviolet A (UVA) radiation. Then the blood with the treated white blood cells is returned to your body.

Retinoids
Retinoids are products related to vitamin A, but can stop the growth of cancer cells. When taken by mouth (orally), they work throughout the body.

Chemotherapy
Chemotherapy kills fast-growing cells throughout the body, including cancer cells and normal cells. All chemotherapies affect the instructions (genes) that tell cancer cells how and when to grow and divide.

Targeted therapy
Targeted therapy focuses on specific or unique features of cancer cells. Targeted therapies seek out how cancer cells grow, divide, and move in the body. These drugs stop the action of molecules that help cancer cells grow and/or survive.

Immunotherapy
Immunotherapy is a targeted therapy that increases the activity of your immune system. By doing so, it improves your body's ability to find and destroy cancer cells. Immunotherapy can be given alone or with other types of treatment.

Warnings!
You might be asked to stop taking or avoid certain herbal supplements when on a systemic therapy. Some supplements can affect the ability of a drug to do its job. This is called a drug interaction. It is critical to speak with your care team about any supplements you may be taking.

Some examples include:

- Turmeric
- Gingko biloba
- Green tea extract
- St. John's Wort

Even certain medicines can affect the ability of a drug to do its job. Antacids, heart medicine, and antidepressants are just some of the medicines that might interact with a systemic therapy. This is why it is important to tell your doctor about any medications, vitamins, over-the-counter (OTC) drugs, herbals, or supplements you are taking. Bring a list with you to every visit.

Clinical trials

Clinical trials study how safe and helpful tests and treatments are for people. Clinical trials find out how to prevent, diagnose, and treat a disease like cancer. Because of clinical trials, scientists and doctors have found, and are continuing to find, new and effective therapies in the management of cancer.

Clinical trials have 4 phases.

- **Phase I trials** aim to find the safest and best dose of a new drug. Another aim is to find the best way to give the drug with the fewest side effects.
- **Phase II trials** assess if a drug works for a specific type of cancer.
- **Phase III trials** formally and scientifically compare a new drug to a standard treatment.
- **Phase IV trials** evaluate a drug's longer term safety and treatment results after it has been approved.

To join a clinical trial, you must meet the conditions of the study. Patients in a clinical trial often are alike in terms of their cancer and general health. This helps to ensure that any change is from the treatment and not because of differences between patients.

If you decide to join a clinical trial, you will need to review and sign a paper called an informed consent form. This form describes the study in detail, including the risks and benefits. Even after you sign a consent form, you can stop taking part in a clinical trial at any time.

Finding a clinical trial

In the U.S.

NCCN Cancer Centers
NCCN.org/cancercenters

The National Cancer Institute (NCI)
cancer.gov/about-cancer/treatment/clinical-trials/search

Worldwide

The U.S. National Library of Medicine (NLM)
clinicaltrials.gov/

Need help finding a clinical trial?
NCI's Cancer Information Service (CIS)

1.800.4.CANCER (1.800.422.6237)

cancer.gov/contact

Ask your treatment team if there is an open clinical trial that you can join. There may be clinical trials where you're getting treatment or at other treatment centers nearby. Discuss the risks and benefits of joining a clinical trial with your care team. Together, decide if a clinical trial is right for you.

3 Treating MF/SS — Stem cell transplant

Stem cell transplant

A stem cell transplant (SCT) replaces bone marrow stem cells. You might hear it called a hematopoietic stem cell transplant (HSCT) or bone marrow transplant (BMT). This book will refer to it as SCT.

There are 2 types:

- Autologous – stem cells come from you
- Allogeneic – stem cells come from a donor that may or may not be related to you

In some cases, an allogeneic SCT (or allo-SCT) is a treatment option. It is used to cure MF/SS. The steps of an allogeneic SCT are described next.

HLA typing

A human leukocyte antigen (HLA) is a protein found on the surface of most cells. It plays an important role in your body's immune response. HLAs are unique to each person. They mark your body's cells. Your body detects these markers to tell which cells are yours. In other words, all your cells have the same set of HLAs. Each person's set of HLAs is called the HLA type or tissue type. HLA type is not dependent on sex or blood group type.

HLA typing is a test that detects a person's HLA type. This test is done before a donor blood stem cell transplant. Your proteins will be compared to the donor's white blood cells to see how many proteins are the same in order to find the best match. A very good match is needed for a transplant to be a treatment option. Otherwise, your body will reject the donor cells or the donor cells will react against your body. Relatives are tested by simple saliva swabs that are sent to them as a kit.

Siblings have a 1 out of 4 (25%) chance of having the same HLA type. If a sibling match cannot be found, then an unrelated match is selected through a registry of volunteer donors. Other donor choices include adult children and parents. Your transplant doctor will select the best match for you.

Conditioning

Before an SCT, treatment is needed to destroy bone marrow cells. This is called conditioning and it creates room for the healthy donor stem cells. It also weakens the immune system so your body won't kill the transplanted cells.

Chemotherapy is used for conditioning. Radiation therapy may also be given as part of conditioning treatment.

Transplanting stem cells

After conditioning, you will receive the healthy stem cells through a transfusion. A transfusion is a slow injection of blood products into a vein. This can take several hours. The transplanted stem cells will travel to your bone marrow and grow. New, healthy blood cells will form. This is called engraftment. It usually takes about 2 to 4 weeks.

Until then, you will have little or no immune defense. You may need to stay in a very clean room at the hospital or be given antibiotics to prevent or treat infection. Transfusions are needed until the new immune system can start making blood component. A red blood cell transfusion is used to prevent bleeding and to treat anemia (below normal red blood cell count). A platelet transfusion is used to treat a low platelet count or bleeding. While waiting for the cells to engraft, you will likely feel tired and weak.

Possible side effects

Every treatment has side effects. You will be monitored for infections, disease relapse, and graft-versus-host disease (GVHD). In GVHD, the donor cells attack your normal, healthy tissue. There are treatments for GVHD. Ask about the possible side effects or complications of SCT and how this might affect your quality of life.

Supportive care

Supportive care is health care that relieves symptoms caused by cancer or its treatment and improves quality of life. It might include pain relief (palliative care), emotional or spiritual support, financial aid, or family counseling. Supportive care is given during all cancer stages. Tell your care team how you are feeling and about any side effects. Best supportive care is used with other treatments to improve quality of life. Best supportive care, supportive care, and palliative care are often used interchangeably.

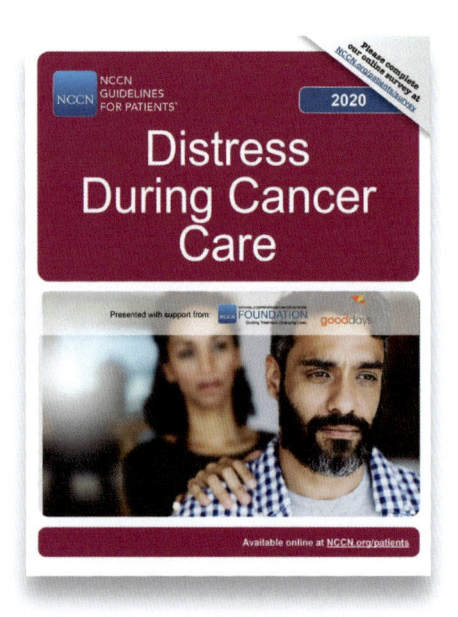

Distress

Distress is an unpleasant experience of a mental, physical, social, or spiritual nature. It can affect how you feel, think, and act. Distress might include feelings of sadness, fear, helplessness, worry, anger, and guilt. You may also experience depression, anxiety, and sleeping problems.

For more information, read *NCCN Guidelines for Patients: Distress During Cancer Care*, available at NCCN.org/patientguidelines.

Itching

Pruritus is very common in those with a cutaneous T-cell lymphoma (CTCL). Pruritus is an itchy feeling that makes you want to scratch your skin. Severe itching may be a side effect of some cancer treatments or a symptom of your cancer. Pruritus sometimes feels like pain. Scratching may cause breaks in the skin, bleeding, and infection. If your skin feels itchy, let your doctor know so it can be treated and relieved. This is important. There are many treatments for pruritus.

Infections

Infections occur frequently in those with MF/SS. Infections of the skin such as bacterial infections and herpes viral infections are common. Tell your care team about any new or worsening symptoms.

Side effects

Because certain therapies directed against destroying cancer cells may also damage healthy cells, many of these therapies may be associated with various side effects.

3 Treating MF/SS | Review

Review

- Treatment decisions should involve a multidisciplinary team (MDT) or a team of doctors from different fields of medicine who have knowledge (expertise) and experience with your type of cancer.

- Skin-directed therapy focuses on the skin and includes topical therapy, local radiation, and phototherapy.

- Systemic therapy works throughout the body. It includes chemotherapy, targeted therapy, immunotherapy, extracorporeal photopheresis (ECP), and retinoids.

- Radiation therapy (RT) uses high-energy radiation from x-rays, protons, gamma rays, and other sources to kill cancer cells and shrink tumors.

- Clinical trials study how safe and helpful tests and cancer treatments are for people.

- An allogeneic stem cell transplant (SCT) uses donor stem cells to replace your bone marrow cells.

- Supportive care is health care that relieves symptoms caused by cancer or its treatment and improves quality of life.

- All cancer treatments can cause unwanted health issues called side effects. You will be monitored for side effects, infection, and other treatment-related issues.

> **Did you know?**
>
> The terms "chemotherapy" and "systemic therapy" are often used interchangeably, but they are not the same. Chemotherapy, targeted therapy, and immunotherapy are all types of systemic therapy.

4
Stage 1A

- 41 Overview
- 41 Primary treatment
- 42 Response to therapy
- 44 Review

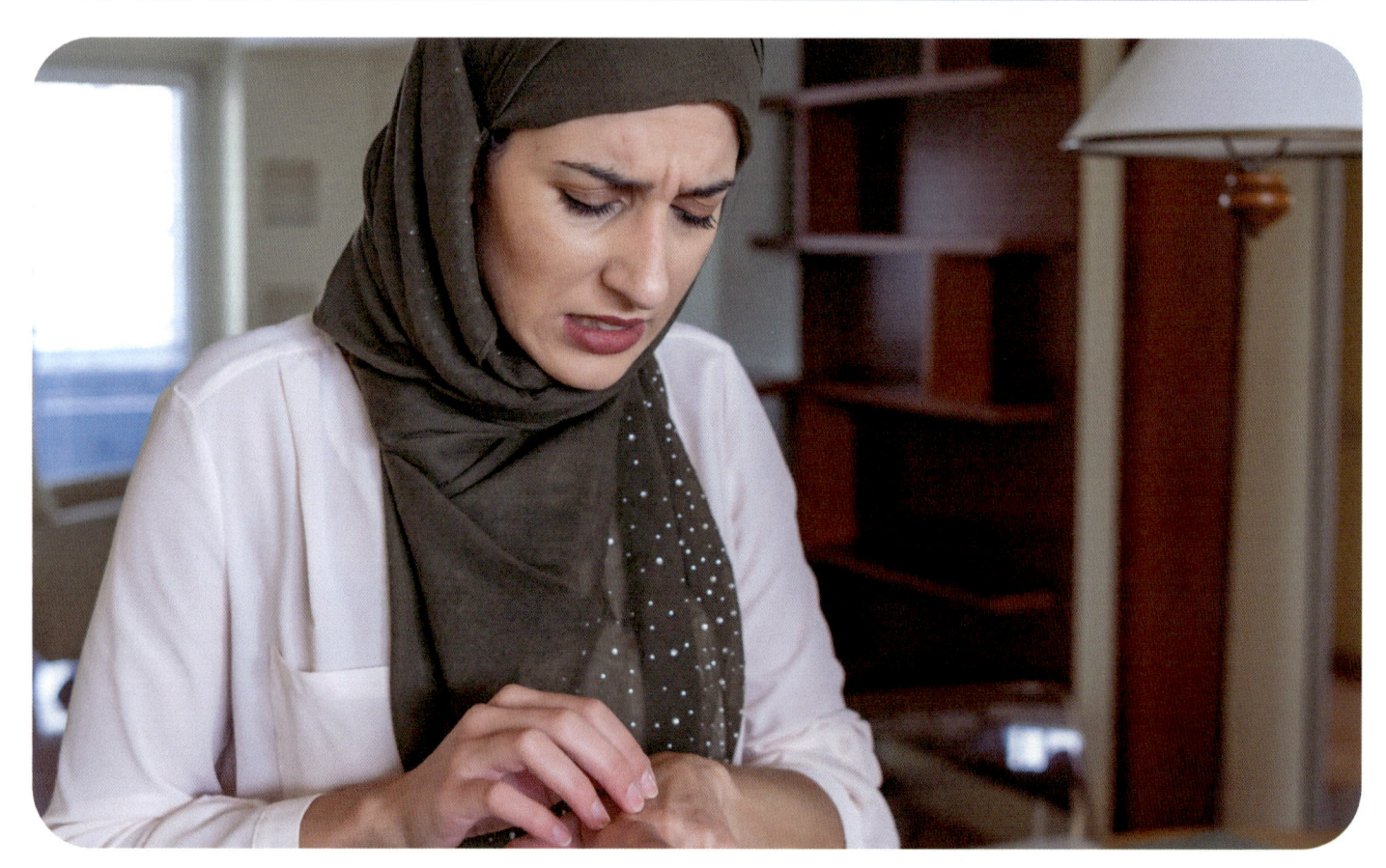

4 Stage 1A | Overview

In stage 1A, cancer is limited to a small area on the skin (T1). Treatment options focus on skin-directed therapies. Together, you and your doctor will choose a treatment plan that is right for you.

Overview

In stage 1A, cancer is limited to a small area on the skin (T1). The amount of cancer is measured by evaluating what percent of your skin is affected by lymphoma. One hand is equal to 1 percent (1%) of your total body surface area (BSA). In stage 1A, less than 10% of the skin (BSA) is covered in patches, papules, and/or plaques.

Primary treatment

Primary treatment is the first treatment tried. Treatment options focus on skin-directed therapies. These therapies may be used alone or with other skin-directed therapies. If abnormal T cells are found in the blood (B1 involvement), then you might be treated for stage 3 (erythrodermic disease).

For skin-directed therapies, see Guide 4.

Guide 4
Skin-directed therapies: Limited or local skin involvement

Local radiation such as involved-site radiation therapy (ISRT)

Phototherapy (UVB or NB-UVB for patch or thin plaques; PUVA or UVA1 for thicker plaques or tumors)

Topical carmustine

Topical corticosteroids

Topical imiquimod

Topical mechlorethamine (nitrogen mustard)

Topical retinoids (bexarotene, tazarotene)

4 Stage 1A | Response to therapy

Response to therapy

Primary treatment aims to improve your condition and to sustain this improvement. A complete response (CR) is described as remission or a disease-free period. In order to maintain remission for as long as possible, maintenance therapy is often given. Maintenance therapy uses the same treatment, but often at a lower dose.

In a partial response (PR), treatment is working, but cancer remains. You will likely continue the same treatment until a CR.

With an inadequate response, the cancer does not seem to respond to current skin-directed therapy. Multiple therapies will be tried to prevent cancer from progressing or spreading.

For treatment options based on response, see Guide 5.

Relapse

When cancer returns after a disease-free period, it is called a relapse. Relapse can happen after a CR or PR.

- If cancer returns and is still T1 skin disease, then treatment will be a skin-directed therapy from Guide 4.
- If cancer returns and it is higher than stage 1A, then the cancer will be restaged. Treatment will be based on the new stage.

Guide 5
Treatment options: Stage 1A (limited skin involvement with less than 10% BSA)

Complete or partial response	If cancer relapse with T1 skin disease, the option is: • Skin-directed therapies (see Guide 4) • Skin-directed therapy may be alone or with other skin-directed therapies
	If cancer relapse with higher-stage disease, then treatment is based on new stage
Inadequate response	If cancer progresses beyond stage 1A on skin-directed therapies, treatment is based on new stage
	If disease refractory to multiple previous therapies, the options are: • Systemic therapy (SYST-CAT A) (see Guide 6) • Systemic therapy (SYST-CAT A) with skin-directed therapy (see Guide 4) • Consider radiation therapy (RT) if not used before • Clinical trial
	If persistent T1 skin disease, options are: • Skin-directed therapies • Consider treatment for stage 3 (erythrodermic disease)

4 Stage 1A | Response to therapy

Progression

Disease progression is cancer that is growing or spreading. If cancer progresses higher than stage 1A, then treatment is based on the new stage.

Persistent

T1 skin disease that persists, but has not progressed, will be treated with a different skin-directed therapy. If cancer in the blood (B1 involvement) is suspected, then treatment will follow stage 3 (erythrodermic disease). Treatment aims to reduce the amount of cancer before starting treatment for refractory disease.

Refractory

When cancer appears resistant to multiple therapies, it is called refractory. Treatment might be systemic therapy with or without skin-directed therapies, radiation therapy if not used before, or a clinical trial.

Systemic therapy at this stage is referred to as systemic therapy category A (SYST-CAT A). These therapies are less toxic than systemic therapies used later in the course of the disease (SYST-CAT B). A preferred treatment is proven to be more effective.

For SYST-CAT A, see Guide 6.

Guide 6
Systemic therapies category A (SYST-CAT A)

Preferred	• Bexarotene • Brentuximab vedotin • Extracorporeal photopheresis (ECP) • Interferons (IFN alfa-2b or IFN gamma-1b) • Methotrexate • Mogamulizumab • Romidepsin • Vorinostat
Other	• Acitretin • All-trans retinoic acid (ATRA) • Isotretinoin (13-cis-retinoic acid)

4 Stage 1A | Review

Review

- In stage 1A, cancer is limited to a small area on the skin (T1). Less than 10% of the skin (BSA) is covered in patches, papules, and/or plaques.

- If abnormal T cells are be found in blood (B1), cancer may be treated as stage 3 erythrodermic disease.

- The goal of treatment is to improve your condition and to sustain this improvement for as long as possible.

- Primary treatment is the first treatment tried. Treatment options focus on skin-directed therapies. These therapies may be used alone or with other skin-directed therapies.

- When cancer returns after a disease-free period, it is called a relapse. Relapse can happen after a complete or partial response.

- Disease progression is cancer that is growing or spreading. If cancer progresses higher than stage 1A, then treatment is based on the new stage.

- Disease that persists will be treated with a different skin-directed therapy.

- When cancer appears resistant to multiple therapies, it is called refractory. Treatment might be systemic therapy (SYST-CAT A) with or without skin-directed therapies, radiation therapy if not used before, or a clinical trial.

> The goal of treatment is to improve your condition and to sustain this improvement for as long as possible.

5
Stage 1B and 2A

46 Overview
47 Low skin disease burden
48 High skin disease burden
50 Review

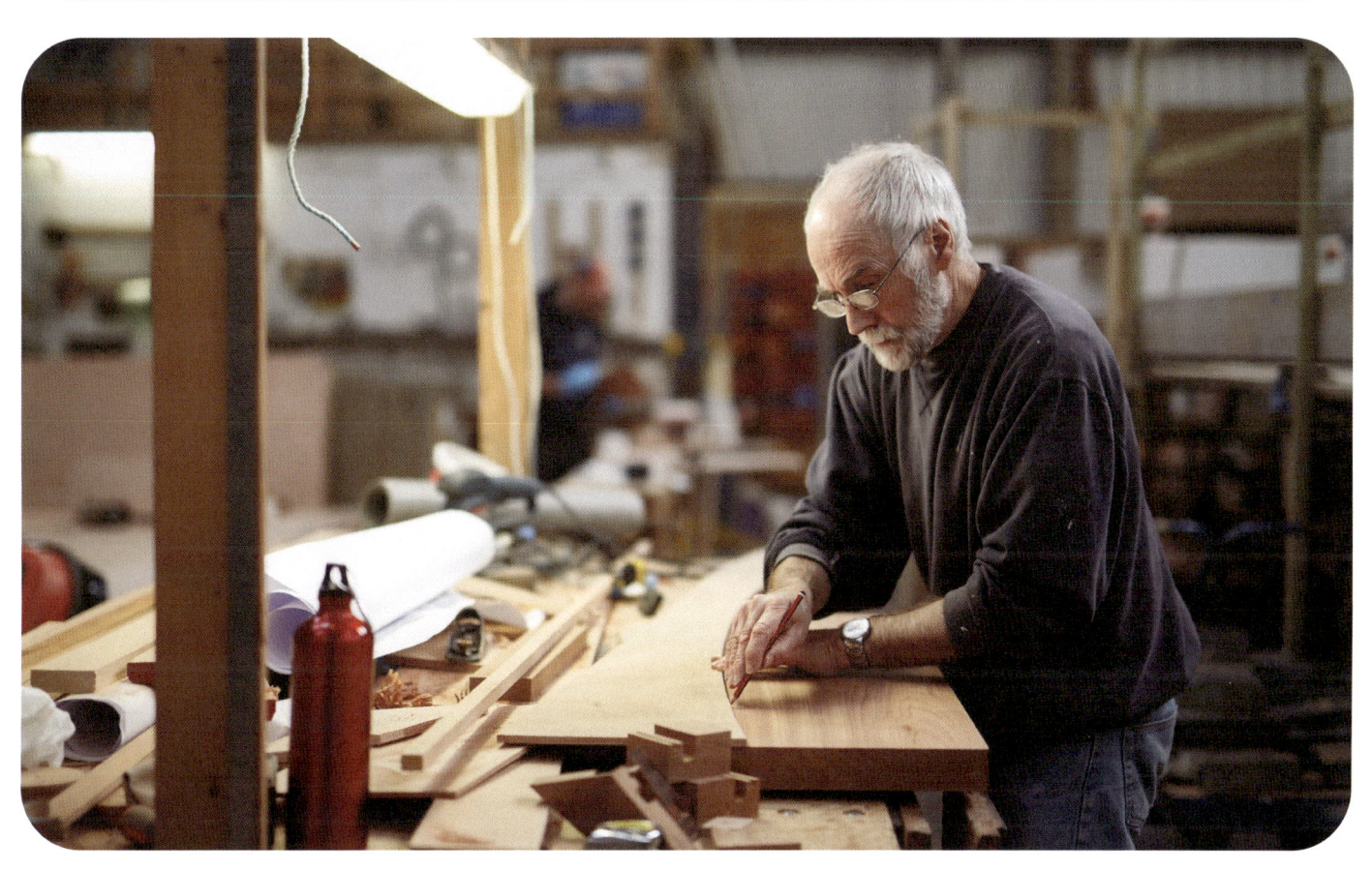

5 Stage 1B and 2A | Overview

Treatment for stage 1B and 2A is based on the amount of skin disease called burden. Low skin disease burden is mostly patch disease. High skin disease burden is mostly plaque disease.

Overview

In stage 1B, patches, papules, and/or plaques cover 10% or more of the skin (T2). Cancer is not found in lymph nodes (N0) or visceral organs (M0). If cancer is found in the blood (B1), it might be treated as stage 3 erythrodermic disease.

In stage 2A, any amount of the skin surface is covered with patches or plaques (T1 or T2). There is no significant involvement (N1 or N2). If cancer is found in the blood (B1), it might be treated as stage 3 erythrodermic disease.

Treatment for stage 1B and 2A is based on the amount of skin disease called burden. The lower the amount of skin disease, the lower the skin disease burden.

Talk to your doctor about which treatment is best for you. Not everyone responds to treatment the same way. Some do better than expected. Others do worse. Your wishes are always important.

Mycosis fungoides

An example of mycosis fungoides skin lesions found on the arm.

Credit: https://commons.wikimedia.org/wiki/File:Mycosis_fungoide.JPG

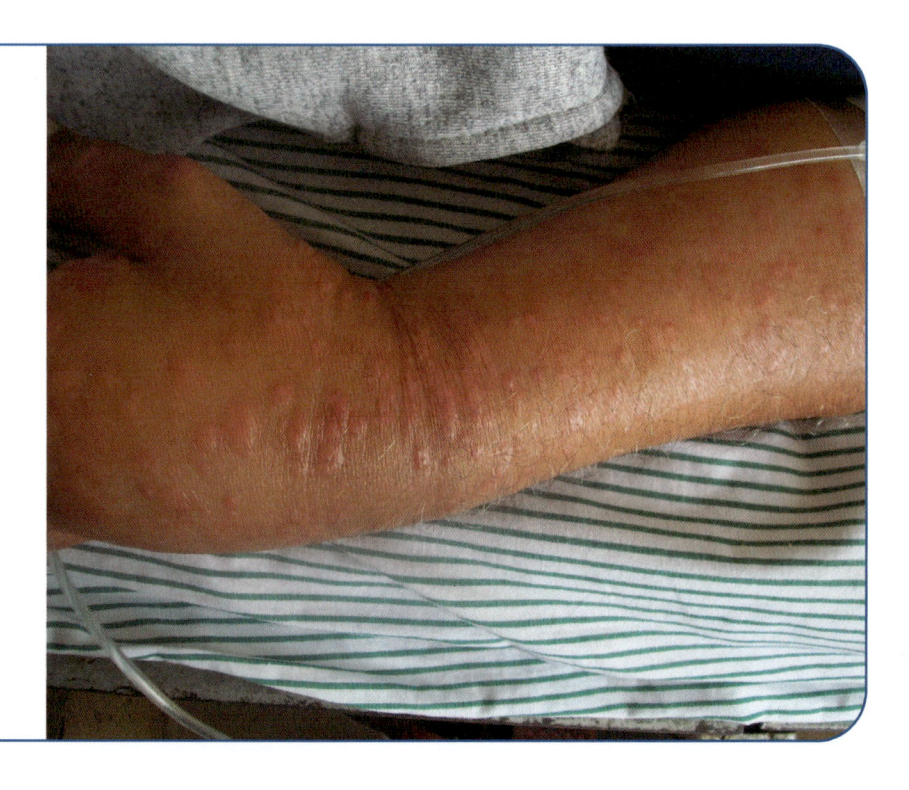

5 Stage 1B and 2A — Low skin disease burden

Low skin disease burden

Low skin disease burden is mostly patch disease. A limited area of the skin is involved. Treatment focuses on limited or local skin-directed therapies. These therapies might be used alone or in combination with other skin-directed therapies. See Guide 7.

Response to therapy

The goal of treatment is to improve your condition and to maintain this improvement for as long as possible. In a complete response (CR) or remission, no signs of disease are found. When cancer returns after a disease-free period, it is called a relapse.

Relapse can happen after a complete or partial response.

- If cancer returns and is still low skin disease burden, then treatment will be a skin-directed therapy.
- If cancer returns and is a high skin disease burden, then treatment will be for high skin disease burden.
- If cancer progresses to higher than stage 1B or 2A, then the cancer will be restaged. Treatment will be based on the new stage.
- If cancer does not respond to treatment, see high skin disease burden treatment options.

Guide 7
Skin-directed therapies

Limited or local skin involvement	• Local radiation such as involved-site radiation therapy (ISRT) • Phototherapy (UVB or NB-UVB for patch or thin plaques; PUVA or UVA1 for thicker plaques or tumors) • Topical carmustine • Topical corticosteroids • Topical imiquimod • Topical mechlorethamine (nitrogen mustard) • Topical retinoids (bexarotene, tazarotene)
General skin involvement	• Phototherapy (UVB or NB-UVB for patch or thin plaques; PUVA or UVA1 for thicker plaques or tumors) • Topical corticosteroids • Topical mechlorethamine (nitrogen mustard) • Total skin electron beam therapy (TSEBT)

5 Stage 1B and 2A | High skin disease burden

High skin disease burden

High skin disease burden is mostly plaque disease. The goal of treatment is to improve your condition and to reduce the amount of cancer burden. If blood (B1 involvement) is suspected, cancer might be treated as stage 3 (erythrodermic disease).

Primary treatment options include:

- Skin-directed therapies for general skin involvement (see Guide 7).
- Systemic therapies (SYST-CAT A) alone or with skin-directed therapies
- Combination therapies alone or with skin-directed therapies

Systemic therapies (SYST-CAT A) can be found in Guide 8.

Combination therapies can include a skin-directed therapy with a systemic therapy or two or more systemic therapies used together. Combination therapies can be found in Guide 9.

Relapse

When cancer returns after a disease-free period, it is called a relapse. Relapse can happen after a complete or partial response.

- If cancer returns and it is T1 or T2 disease, then the same or another primary treatment option might be given.
- If cancer returns and it is higher than stage 1B or 2A, then the cancer will be restaged. Treatment will be based on the new stage.

Guide 8
Systemic therapies category A (SYST-CAT A)

Preferred	• Bexarotene • Brentuximab vedotin • Extracorporeal photopheresis (ECP) • Interferons (IFN alfa-2b or IFN gamma-1b) • Methotrexate • Mogamulizumab • Romidepsin • Vorinostat
Other	• Acitretin • All-trans retinoic acid (ATRA) • Isotretinoin (13-cis-retinoic acid)

5 Stage 1B and 2A | High skin disease burden

Progression
If cancer progresses to higher than stage 1B or 2A, then the cancer will be restaged. Treatment will be based on the new stage.

Persistent
Persistent is disease that remains after completing primary treatment. Persistent T1 or T2 disease should be treated with a primary treatment option not received before. The aim is to reduce the amount of cancer before choosing a treatment for refractory disease.

Refractory
When cancer appears resistant to multiple therapies, it is called refractory.

Treatment options include:

- Clinical trial
- Total skin electron beam therapy (TSEBT), if not used before
- Combination therapies with or without skin-directed therapy

Guide 9
Combination therapy options

Skin-directed with systemic therapy	• Phototherapy with extracorporeal photopheresis (ECP) • Phototherapy with interferon (IFN alfa-2b or IFN gamma-1b) • Phototherapy with a retinoid • Total skin electron beam therapy (TSEBT) with ECP
Systemic therapy with systemic therapy	• ECP with interferon (IFN alfa-2b or IFN gamma-1b) • ECP with a retinoid • ECP with a retinoid and interferon (IFN alfa-2b or IFN gamma-1b) • Retinoid with interferon (IFN alfa-2b or IFN gamma-1b)

Review

- Treatment for stage 1B and 2A is based on the amount of skin disease called burden. The lower the amount of skin disease, the lower the skin disease burden.

- Low skin disease burden is mostly patch disease. Treatment focuses on skin-directed therapies.

- High skin disease burden is mostly plaque disease. Treatment options include skin-directed therapies, systemic therapies (SYST-CAT A), and combination therapies.

- The goal of primary treatment is to improve your condition and to reduce the amount of cancer burden.

- A disease-free period is called remission or complete response (CR). When cancer returns after a disease-free period, it is called a relapse. Relapse can happen after a complete or partial response (PR).

- Persistent is disease that remains after completing primary treatment. A different primary treatment will be tried.

- When cancer appears resistant to multiple therapies, it is called refractory.

6
Stage 2B

52	**Overview**
52	**Limited tumors**
53	**Widespread tumors**
55	**Review**

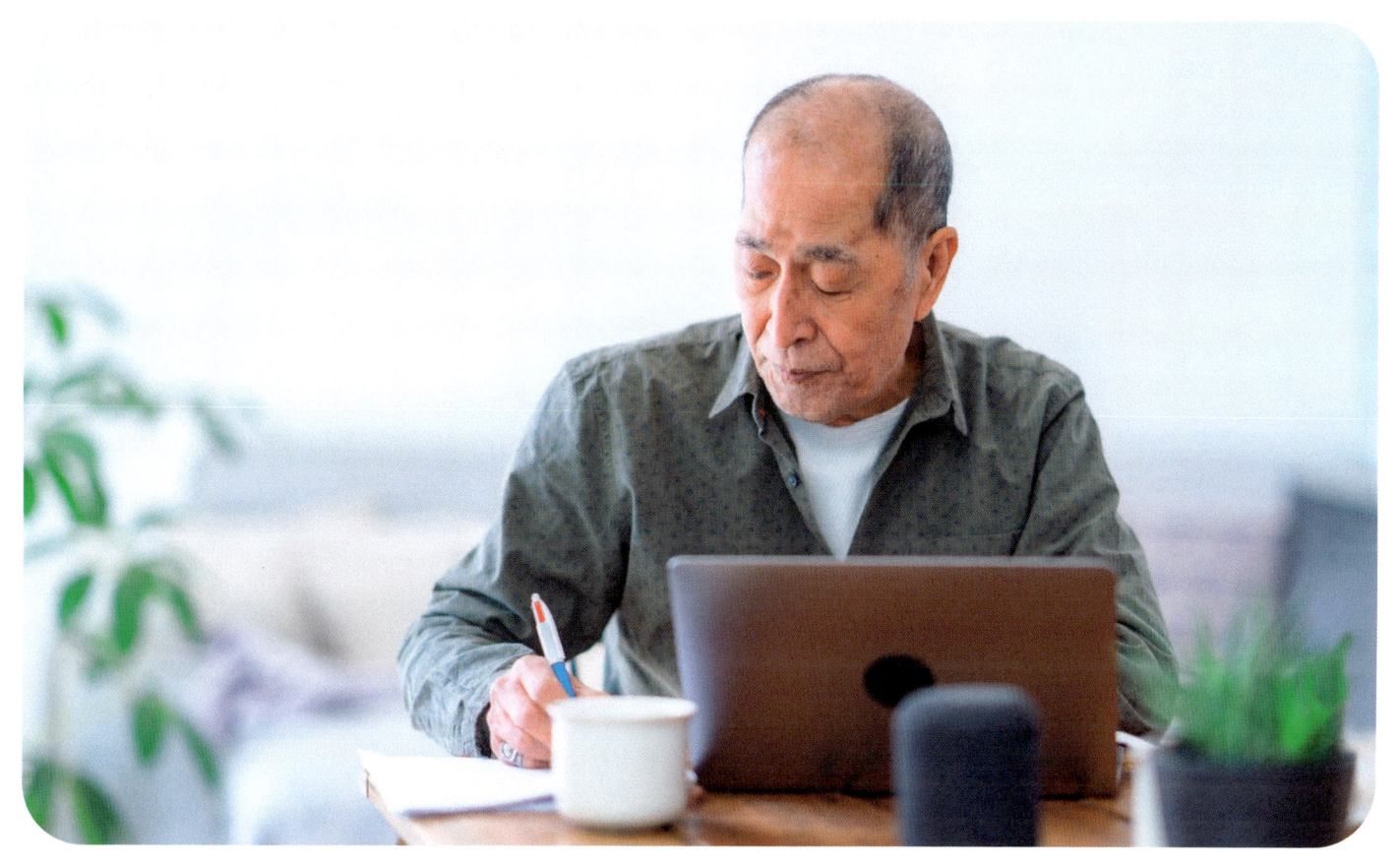

6 Stage 2B | Overview

Stage 2B is also called tumor stage disease. Treatment is based on if the tumors are limited or widespread. Together, you and your doctor will choose a treatment plan that is right for you.

Overview

Stage 2B is also called tumor stage disease. In this stage, one or more tumors 1 cm or more in size are found on the skin. Treatment is based on if the tumors are limited or widespread. Abnormal T cells may be found in the lymph nodes and/or blood.

Limited tumors

Primary treatment
Primary treatment is the first treatment. The goal of treatment is to improve your condition and to sustain this improvement.

Primary treatment options include:

- Local radiation therapy (RT) and/or skin-directed therapies
- Systemic therapies (SYST-CAT A) with or without local RT
- Local RT is preferred for tumor lesions

Relapse
When cancer returns after a disease-free period, it is called a relapse. Relapse can happen after a complete or partial response to primary treatment.

If cancer returns and it is:

- T1 disease, then it will be treated as stage 1A
- T2 disease, then it will be treated as stage 1B and 2A
- Limited T3 disease, then the same or another primary treatment option might be given
- Higher than stage 2B, then the cancer will be restaged. Treatment will be based on the new stage.

Progression
If cancer spreads or advances to a stage higher than 2B, then the cancer will be restaged. Treatment will be based on the new stage.

Persistent
Persistent is disease that remains after completing primary treatment. Persistent T1, T2, or T3 with widespread tumor lesions should be treated with the other primary treatment options not received before. The aim is to reduce the amount of cancer before choosing a treatment for refractory disease.

Refractory
When cancer appears resistant to multiple therapies, it is called refractory. Treatment will follow widespread tumors described next.

6 Stage 2B | Widespread tumors

Widespread tumors

Primary treatment
Primary treatment is the first treatment. The goal is to reduce the amount of cancer in the body and to prevent further spread.

Treatment options include:

- Total skin electron beam therapy (TSEBT)
- Systemic therapies (SYST-CAT A)
- Systemic therapies (SYST-CAT B)
- Combination therapies
- Skin-directed therapy might be used with systemic or combination therapies

In general, SYST-CAT A options will be considered first before moving on to SYST-CAT B options. SYST-CAT A therapies are less toxic than SYST-CAT B therapies.

Relapse
When cancer returns after a disease-free period, it is called a relapse. Relapse can happen after a complete or partial response.

If cancer returns and it is:

- T1 disease, then it will be treated as stage 1A
- T2 disease, then it will be treated as stage 1B and 2A
- Limited T3 disease, then the same or another primary treatment option might be given
- Higher than stage 2B, then the cancer will be restaged. Treatment will be based on the new stage

SYST-CAT A

Systemic category A (SYST-CAT A) therapies will be tried before SYST-CAT B therapies.

Preferred options
- Bexarotene
- Brentuximab vedotin
- Extracorporeal photopheresis (ECP)
- Interferons (IFN alfa-2b or IFN gamma-1b)
- Methotrexate
- Mogamulizumab
- Romidepsin
- Vorinostat

Other options
- Acitretin
- All-trans retinoic acid
- Isotretinoin (13-cis-retinoic acid)

SYST-CAT B

Preferred options
- Brentuximab vedotin
- Gemcitabine
- Liposomal doxorubicin
- Pralatrexate

6 Stage 2B — Widespread tumors

Progression
If cancer spreads or advances to a stage higher than 2B, then the cancer will be restaged. Treatment will be based on the new stage.

Persistent
Persistent is disease that remains after completing primary treatment. Persistent T1 to T3 with widespread tumor lesions disease should be treated with the other primary treatment options not received before. The goal is to improve response before moving on to treatment for refractory disease.

Refractory
When cancer appears resistant to multiple therapies, it is called refractory.

Treatment options include:

- Systemic therapy if large-cell transformation (LCT)
- Systemic therapy for relapsed or refractory disease (see Guide 10)
- Clinical trial
- Allogeneic SCT (allo-SCT)

An allo-SCT is not an option for everyone. LCT can happen at any stage and is identified by the presence of large cells. If LCT is found, it will be treated in addition to mycosis fungoides.

For LCT, the preferred options are:

- Brentuximab vedotin
- Gemcitabine
- Liposomal doxorubicin
- Pralatrexate
- Romidepsin

Guide 10
Systemic therapy options: Relapsed or refractory disease (in some cases)

Alemtuzumab
Chlorambucil
Cyclophosphamide
Etoposide
Pembrolizumab
Pentostatin
Temozolomide for central nervous system (CNS) involvement
Bortezomib

6 Stage 2B | Review

Review

- Stage 2B is also called tumor stage disease. Treatment is based on if the tumors are limited or widespread.

- The goal of primary treatment is to improve your condition and to reduce the amount of disease.

- When cancer returns after a disease-free period, it is called a relapse. Relapse can happen after a complete or partial response (PR).

- If cancer spreads or advances to a stage higher than 2B, then the cancer will be restaged. Treatment will be based on the new stage.

- When cancer appears resistant to multiple therapies, it is called refractory.

- Large-cell transformation (LCT) can happen at any stage. If LCT is found, it will be treated in addition to mycosis fungoides.

> Participation in a clinical trial is recommended for those with refractory disease.

7
Stage 3

57 **Primary treatment**
58 **Response to therapy**
59 **Review**

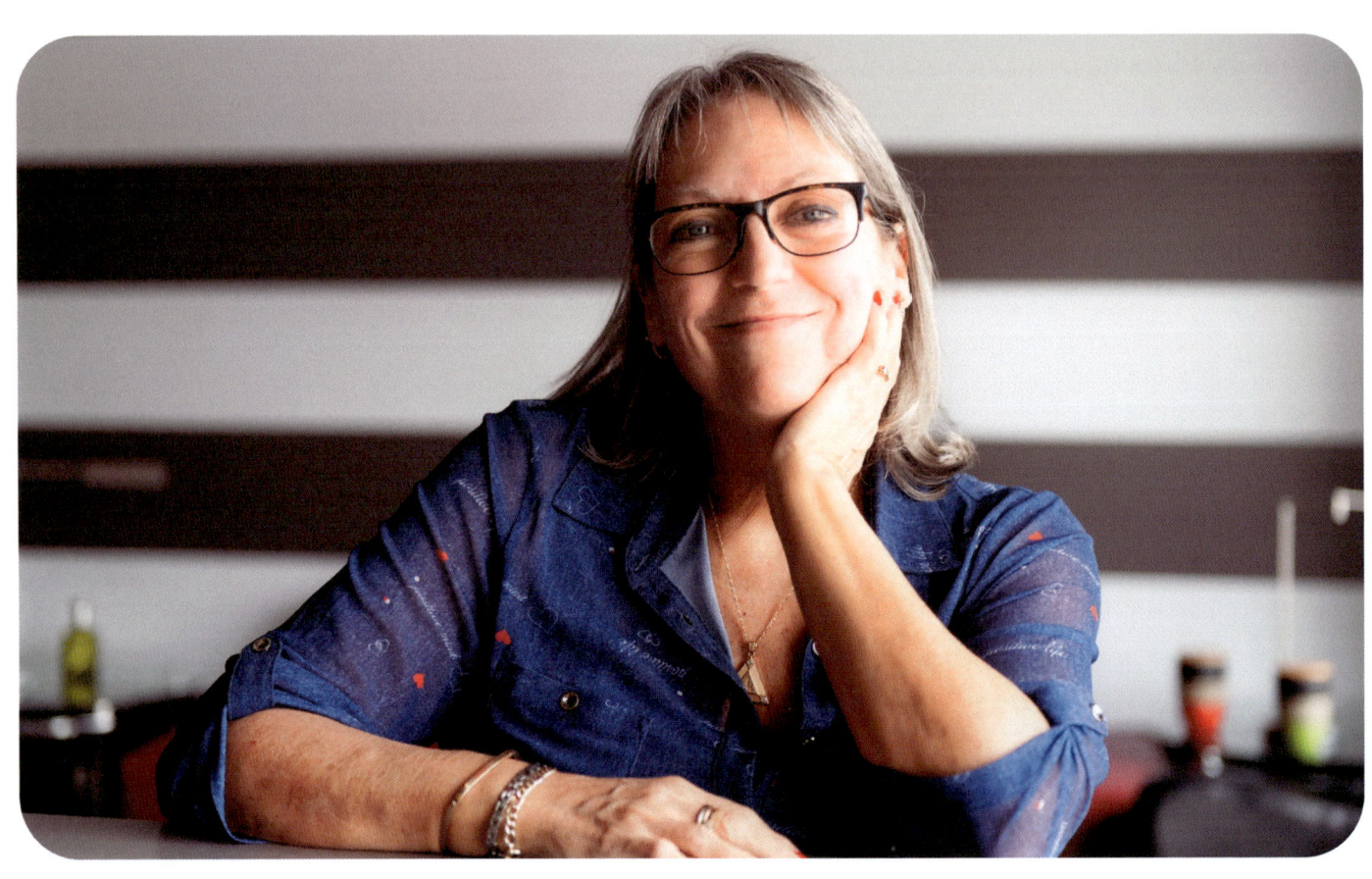

7 Stage 3 | Primary treatment

Stage 3 is also called erythrodermic disease. In erythrodermic disease, nearly all of the skin is reddened (erythema). Cancer may be in lymph nodes (any N) or blood (B1).

Primary treatment

Primary treatment is the first treatment tried. Options described below are based on low or intermediate disease burden. Ask about your level of disease burden and how this might affect treatment options.

Preferred treatment options for low or intermediate disease burden include:

- Combination therapies (see Guide 11)
- SYST-CAT A alone or with skin-directed therapies

Other options include:

- SYST-CAT B alone or with skin-directed therapies
- Alemtuzumab
- Pembrolizumab

Since erythroderma covers most of the body, skin-directed therapies will be for general skin involvement. These include phototherapy, topical corticosteroids, topical mechlorethamine, and total skin electron beam therapy (TSEBT).

Guide 11
Combination therapy options

Skin-directed with systemic therapy	• Phototherapy with extracorporeal photopheresis (ECP) • Phototherapy with interferon (IFN alfa-2b or IFN gamma-1b) • Phototherapy with a retinoid • Total skin electron beam therapy (TSEBT) with ECP
Systemic therapy with systemic therapy	• ECP with interferon (IFN alfa-2b or IFN gamma-1b) • ECP with a retinoid • ECP with a retinoid and interferon (IFN alfa-2b or IFN gamma-1b) • Retinoid with interferon (IFN alfa-2b or IFN gamma-1b)

7　Stage 3 | Response to therapy

Response to therapy

The goal of treatment is to improve your condition and to maintain this improvement for as long as possible. When cancer returns after a disease-free period, it is called a relapse. Relapse can happen after a complete or partial response.

Relapse
If cancer returns and is still low or intermediate disease burden, then the same primary treatment might be used again.

Progression
If cancer progresses to stage 4, then cancer will follow stage 4 treatment options.

Persistent
Persistent disease should be treated with the other primary treatment options not received before.

Refractory
When cancer appears resistant to multiple therapies, it is called refractory. Treatment aims to control or reduce the amount of cancer burden in the body.

Treatment options include:

> Clinical trial

> Systemic therapy for high disease burden (see Guide 12) or relapsed/refractory disease (see Guide 10)

> Allogeneic stem cell transplant (allo-SCT)

Not everyone is a candidate for an allo-SCT. Discuss with your doctor which options might be right for you. Your wishes are always important.

Guide 12
Erythrodermic disease systemic therapy options: High disease burden

Preferred	• Combination therapy options (see Guide 11) • Mogamulizumab alone or with skin-directed therapies (skin-generalized) • Romidepsin alone or with skin-directed therapies (skin-generalized)
Other	• SYST-CAT A (options not listed under preferred) • SYST-CAT B • Alemtuzumab • Pembrolizumab

NCCN Guidelines for Patients®
Mycosis Fungoides/Sézary Syndrome, 2021

Review

- Stage 3 is also called erythrodermic disease. In erythrodermic disease, nearly all of the skin is reddened (erythema).

- Blood tumor burden is based on the number of abnormal T cells found in the blood.

- The goal of treatment is to improve your condition and to maintain this improvement for as long as possible.

- When cancer returns after a disease-free period, it is called a relapse. Relapse can happen after a complete (CR) or partial response (PR).

- If cancers spreads or advances to another stage, then treatment is based on the new stage.

- Persistent disease does not seem to be responding to treatment. If this is the case, a different primary treatment option will be tried.

- When cancer appears resistant to multiple therapies, it is called refractory. Treatment might be a clinical trial, systemic therapy, or an allogeneic SCT (allo-SCT). Not everyone is a candidate for an allo-SCT.

8
Stage 4

61	**Overview**
62	**Sézary syndrome**
63	**Non-Sézary disease**
64	**Visceral disease**
65	**Review**

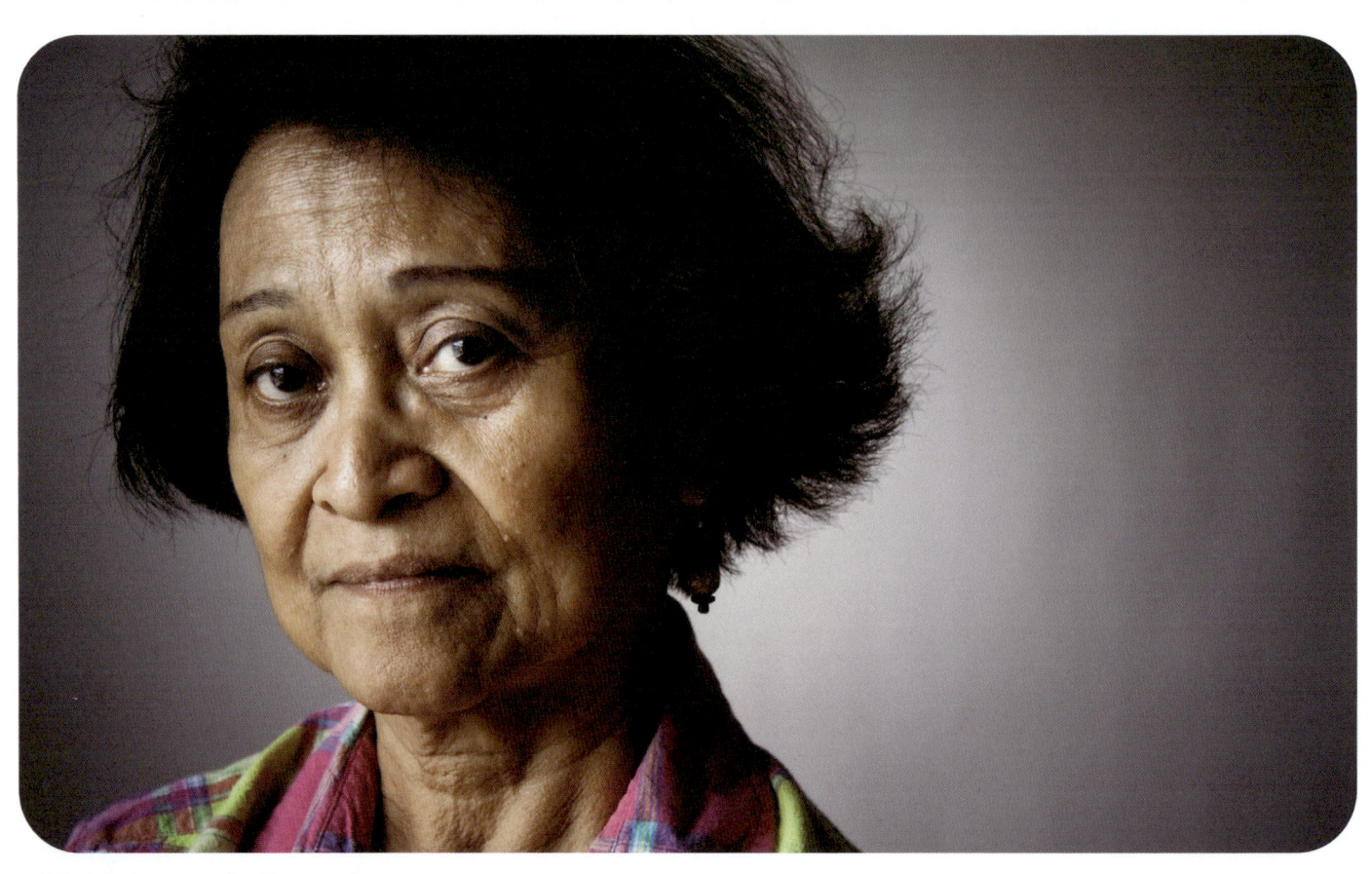

8 Stage 4 | Overview

Stage 4 includes Sézary syndrome (stage $4A_1$ or $4A_2$), non-Sézary disease (stage $4A_2$), and visceral disease (stage 4B). Treatment options include systemic therapy, skin-directed therapies, clinical trial, or stem cell transplant.

In Sézary syndrome a widespread red rash called erythroderma covers most of the body. Erythroderma is caused by abnormal T cells called Sézary cells. These cells can be found in the skin, blood, and lymph nodes. Enlarged lymph nodes (lymphadenopathy) are also common.

Sézary syndrome uses the same staging system as mycosis fungoides.

Overview

Stage 4 is divided into:

- Sézary syndrome (stage $4A_1$ or $4A_2$)
- Non-Sézary (stage $4A_2$) or visceral disease (stage 4B)

Erythroderma

Erythroderma is severe inflammation of most of the body's skin surface. It can look like sunburn or large splotches.

Credit: https://commons.wikimedia.org/wiki/File:Sezery2.jpg

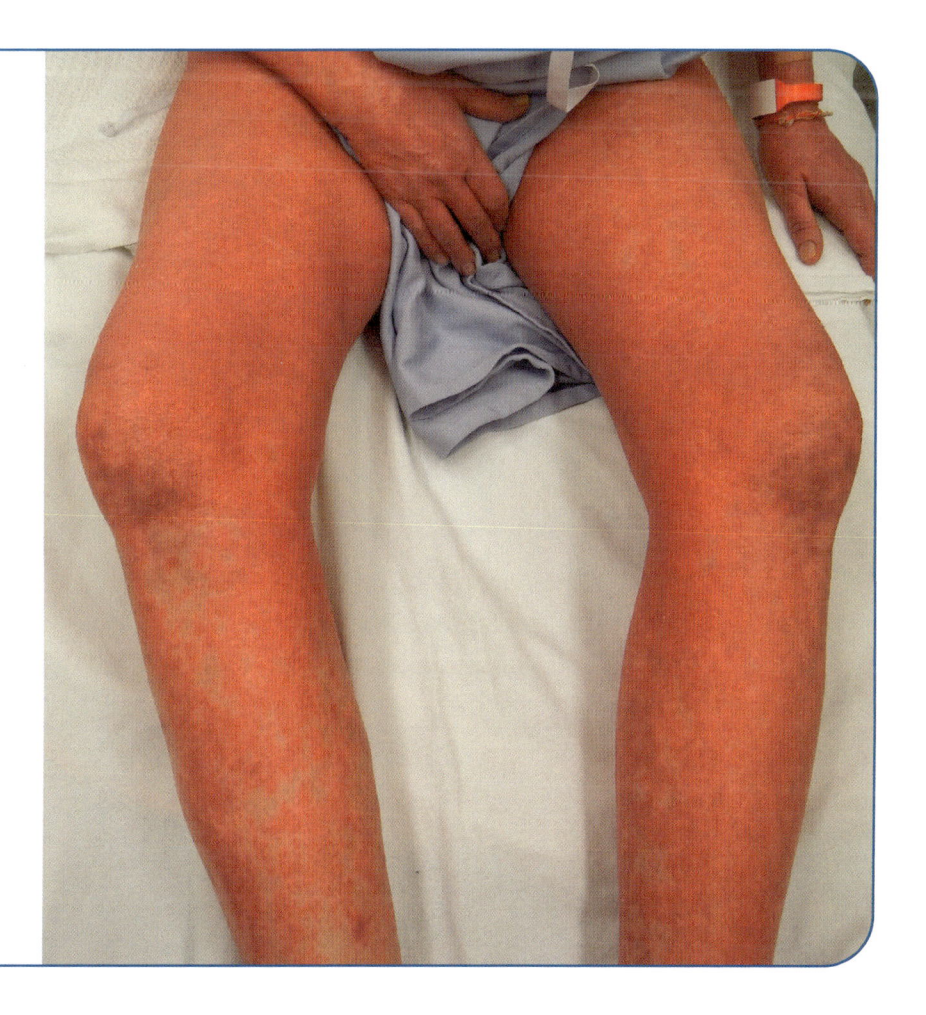

8 Stage 4 — Sézary syndrome

Sézary syndrome

Sézary syndrome (SS) is stage 4A1 and 4A2. Skin can be any stage (any T). Cancer may be found in lymph nodes and/or blood (B2). A diagnosis of SS requires B2 involvement.

Primary treatment is based on whether disease burden is low or high. Burden refers to the amount of disease. The goal of treatment is to reduce disease burden.

For low to intermediate disease burden, see Guide 13.

For high disease burden, see Guide 14.

Relapse
When cancer returns after a disease-free period, it is called a relapse. Relapse can happen after a complete or partial response. Treatment is based on the disease burden discussed on the previous page.

Persistent
Persistent disease following completion of primary treatment should be treated with the other primary treatment options not received before to improve response before moving on to treatment for refractory disease.

Guide 13
Sézary syndrome: Low or intermediate disease burden

Preferred	• Combination therapies (see Guide 11) • SYST-CAT A alone or with skin-directed therapies (skin-generalized)
Other	• SYST-CAT B alone or with skin-directed therapies (skin-generalized) • Alemtuzumab • Pembrolizumab

Guide 14
Sézary syndrome options: High disease burden

Preferred	• Combination therapies (see Guide 11) • Mogamulizumab alone or with skin-directed therapies (skin-generalized) • Romidepsin alone or with skin-directed therapies (skin-generalized)
Other	• SYST-CAT A (options not listed under preferred) • SYST-CAT B • Alemtuzumab • Pembrolizumab

8 Stage 4 — Non-Sézary disease

Non-Sézary disease

In non-Sézary stage 4A2 disease, skin can be any stage (any T). Abnormal T lymphocytes have altered the structure of lymph nodes (N3). Cancer may be found in blood.

Primary treatment

Primary treatment is the first treatment. Primary treatment aims to improve your condition and to sustain this improvement.

Treatment options:

- Systemic therapies (SYST-CAT B)
- Systemic therapies for large-cell transformation (LCT)
- Radiation therapy might be added

After a complete or partial response, treatment might be from the list above, clinical trial, or allogeneic stem cell transplant (allo-SCT). An allo-SCT is not for everyone. Persistent disease will be treated with another primary treatment.

Preferred SYST-CAT B options:

- Brentuximab vedotin
- Gemcitabine
- Liposomal doxorubicin
- Pralatrexate

Large-cell transformation

Large-cell transformation (LCT) can happen at any stage and is identified by the presence of large cells. If LCT is found, it will be treated in addition to mycosis fungoides.

For LCT preferred options, see Guide 15.

Guide 15
Systemic therapy options: Large-cell transformation (LCT)

Brentuximab vedotin
Gemcitabine
Liposomal doxorubicin
Pralatrexate
Romidepsin

8 Stage 4 | Visceral disease

Visceral disease

Visceral disease is cancer that has spread or metastasized to a solid organ such as the spleen or liver. Imaging tests will be used to confirm visceral disease and might be used to see how your body is responding to treatment.

In stage 4B, cancer has metastasized (M1) to internal (visceral) organs. Skin can be any stage (any T). Lymph nodes and blood can be any stage (any N, any B).

Both mycosis fungoides (MF) and Sézary syndrome (SS) can be stage 4B visceral disease. Treatment is systemic therapy alone or with radiation therapy. Systemic therapy works throughout the body to reduce the amount of cancer in the organs and blood. It includes retinoids, chemotherapy, targeted therapy, and immunotherapy. Radiation therapy might be used to treat skin lesions.

If large-cell transformation (LCT) is suspected, you might have a biopsy. LCT occurs when a specific group of MF tumor cells undergo molecular and/or genetic changes that cause them to become larger. LCT will be treated in addition to MF.

Primary treatment

Primary treatment aims to improve your condition and to sustain this improvement. A complete response (CR) is described as remission or a disease-free period.

Primary treatment options:

- Systemic therapies (SYST-CAT B)
- Systemic therapies for LCT
- Radiation therapy might be added

Relapse

When cancer returns after a disease-free period, it is called a relapse. Relapse can happen after a complete or partial response. Treatment will be a clinical trial or allogeneic stem cell transplant (allo-SCT). An allo-SCT is not for everyone. Ask if another relapse is possible and how treatment might affect future options.

Persistent

Persistent disease following completion of primary treatment should be treated with a different systemic therapy from the primary treatments listed above. The goal is to improve response before moving on to treatment for refractory disease. Multiple primary treatments might be tried.

Refractory

When cancer appears resistant to multiple therapies, it is called refractory. Treatment options are the same for all stage 4 refractory disease.

Treatment options:

- Clinical trial
- Systemic therapy
- Allogeneic SCT

An allo-SCT is not for everyone. Ask your doctor which option might be best for your type of MF/SS. Your wishes are always important.

Review

- In Sézary syndrome (SS), cancerous T cells called Sézary cells are found in the skin, lymph nodes, and blood.

- Visceral disease is cancer that has spread or metastasized to a solid organ such as the spleen or liver.

- Imaging tests will be used to confirm visceral disease and might be used to see how your body is responding to treatment.

- In stage 4B, cancer has metastasized (M1) to internal (visceral) organs. Skin can be any stage (any T). Lymph nodes and blood can be any stage (any N, any B).

- When cancer appears resistant to multiple therapies, it is called refractory. Treatment options are the same for all stage 4 refractory disease.

> In Sézary syndrome, a widespread rash called erythroderma covers most of the body.

9
Large-cell transformation

67 Overview
67 Limited lesions with LCT
69 Widespread lesions with LCT
69 Review

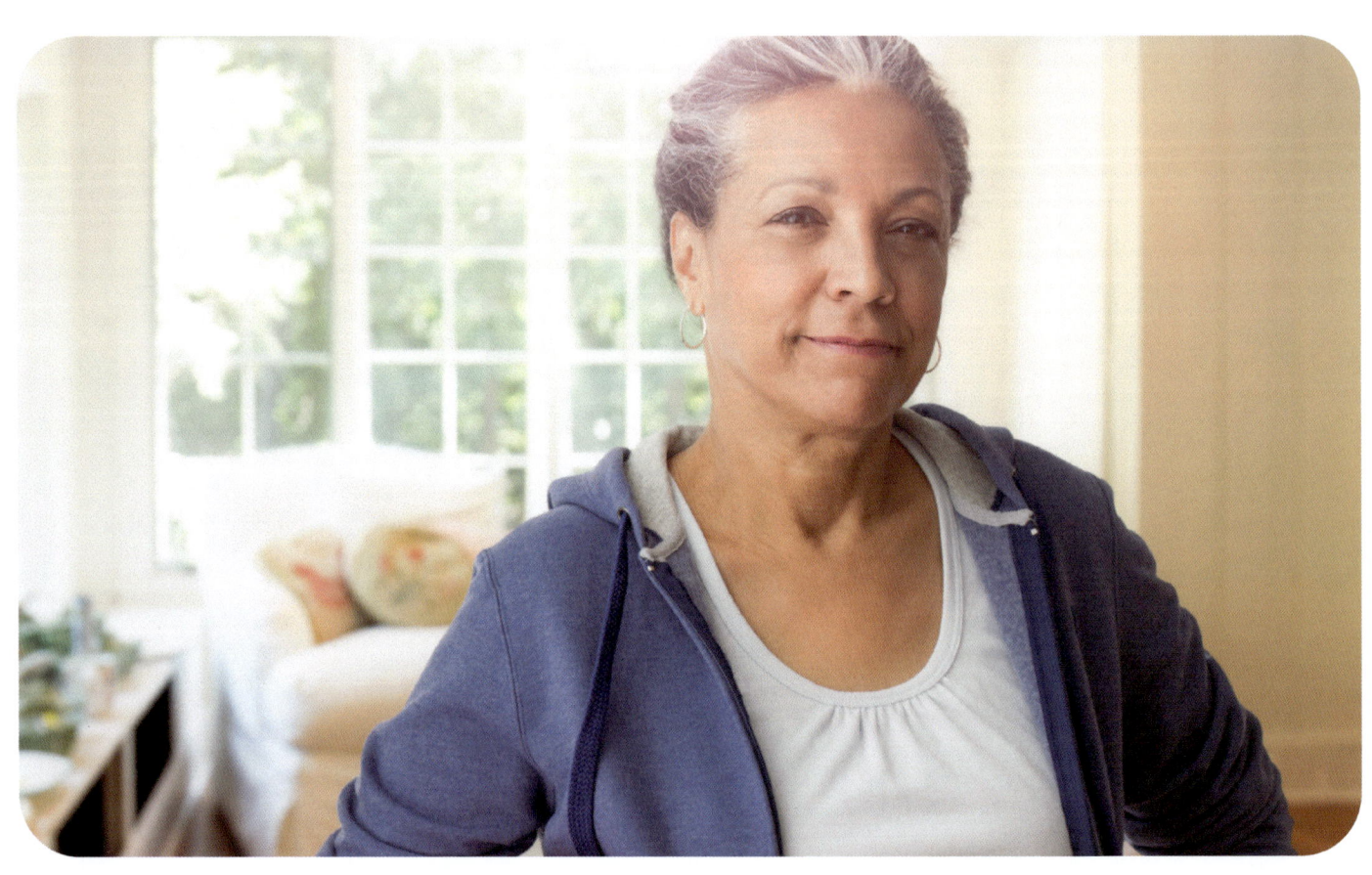

9 Large-cell transformation | Overview

Large-cell transformation (LCT) occurs when a specific group of mycosis fungoides (MF) tumor cells undergo molecular and/or genetic changes that cause them to become larger. Both LCT and MF will be treated. LCT will be treated based on the number of lesions with LCT. MF will be treated based on the cancer stage.

Overview

Large-cell transformation (LCT) is diagnosed when large cells are present in more than 25 percent (25%) of tumor cells in a skin lesion biopsy. This means that a large cell is found in more than 1 out of every 4 tumor cells. Typically, mycosis fungoides (MF) grows and progresses slowly, but sometimes it transforms in LCT and may become more aggressive. This can occur in any stage.

Both LCT and MF will be treated. Treatment directed at LCT aims to slow the growth of LCT. At the same time, MF will be treated to prevent the cancer stage from advancing. Treatment for LCT is described next. Treatment for MF stages can be found in previous chapters.

Limited lesions with LCT

If there are a limited number of lesions with LCT, the lesions might be treated with radiation therapy. Treatment for MF will continue based on cancer stage. The goal of treatment is to improve your condition and to maintain this improvement for as long as possible.

In a complete response (CR) or remission, no signs of disease are found. In a partial response (PR), treatment is working, but cancer remains. You will likely continue the same treatment after a PR.

With an inadequate response, cancer does not seem to be responding to current treatment. Multiple therapies will be tried to prevent cancer from progressing or spreading. Imaging and other tests might be performed if disease is suspected in lymph nodes and/or internal (visceral) organs.

Relapse
When cancer returns after a disease-free period, it is called a relapse. Relapse can happen after a complete or partial response. Treatment might the same as used before. LCT lesions might be treated with radiation therapy. Treatment for MF will be based on cancer stage.

Persistent
In LCT that persists, but has not progressed, treatment will continue to focus on both LCT and MF. The aim is to reduce the amount of cancer before choosing a treatment for refractory disease.

9 Large-cell transformation | Limited lesions with LCT

Refractory

When cancer appears resistant to multiple therapies, it is called refractory. Treatment might be systemic therapy, an allogeneic stem cell transplant (allo-SCT), or a clinical trial. Treatment will continue to focus on both diseases.

LCT systemic therapy options are:

- Brentuximab vedotin
- Gemcitabine
- Liposomal doxorubicin
- Pralatrexate
- Romidepsin

For relapsed or refractory systemic therapy options, see Guide 16.

> Large-cell transformation (LCT) will be treated in addition to mycosis fungoides (MF).

Guide 16
Systemic therapy options: Relapsed or refractory disease
Alemtuzumab
Chlorambucil
Cyclophosphamide
Etoposide
Pembrolizumab
Pentostatin
Temozolomide for central nervous system (CNS) involvement
Bortezomib

9 Large-cell transformation | Widespread lesions with LCT | Review

Widespread lesions with LCT

This section is for widespread skin lesions with LCT. It also includes lesions with LCT found in organs. Treatment includes systemic therapy with or without skin-directed therapy. The systemic therapy will help control LCT that is found in any organs and skin lesions. Treatment will continue for MF as well.

The goal of primary treatment is to slow the growth of LCT. Imaging and other tests might be performed if disease is suspected in lymph nodes and/or internal (visceral) organs.

Complete or partial response
When cancer returns after a disease-free period, it is called a relapse. Relapse can happen after a complete or partial response.

Treatment options include:

- LCT systemic therapy with or without skin-directed therapy
- Clinical trial
- Allogeneic SCT

Persistent
In LCT that persists, but has not progressed, treatment will continue to focus on both LCT and MF. It will include LCT systemic therapy used alone or with skin-directed therapy. The goal is reduce the amount of cancer before starting treatment for refractory disease.

Refractory
When cancer appears resistant to multiple therapies, it is called refractory. Treatment might be clinical trial, systemic therapy, or allogeneic stem cell transplant (allo-SCT).

Review

- Large-cell transformation (LCT) occurs when a specific group of mycosis fungoides (MF) tumor cells undergo molecular and/or genetic changes that cause them to become larger.
- LCT is diagnosed when large cells are present in more than 25 percent (25%) of tumor cells in a skin lesion biopsy. This means that a large cell is found in more than 1 out of every 4 MF cells.
- LCT will be treated in addition to MF. Treatment for LCT is based on the number of lesions with LCT. Treatment for MF will be based on the cancer stage.
- LCT can happen in any MF stage.
- A clinical trial or allogeneic stem cell transplant (allo-SCT) might be an option in some cases.

10
Making treatment decisions

71 It's your choice
71 Questions to ask your doctors
82 Resources

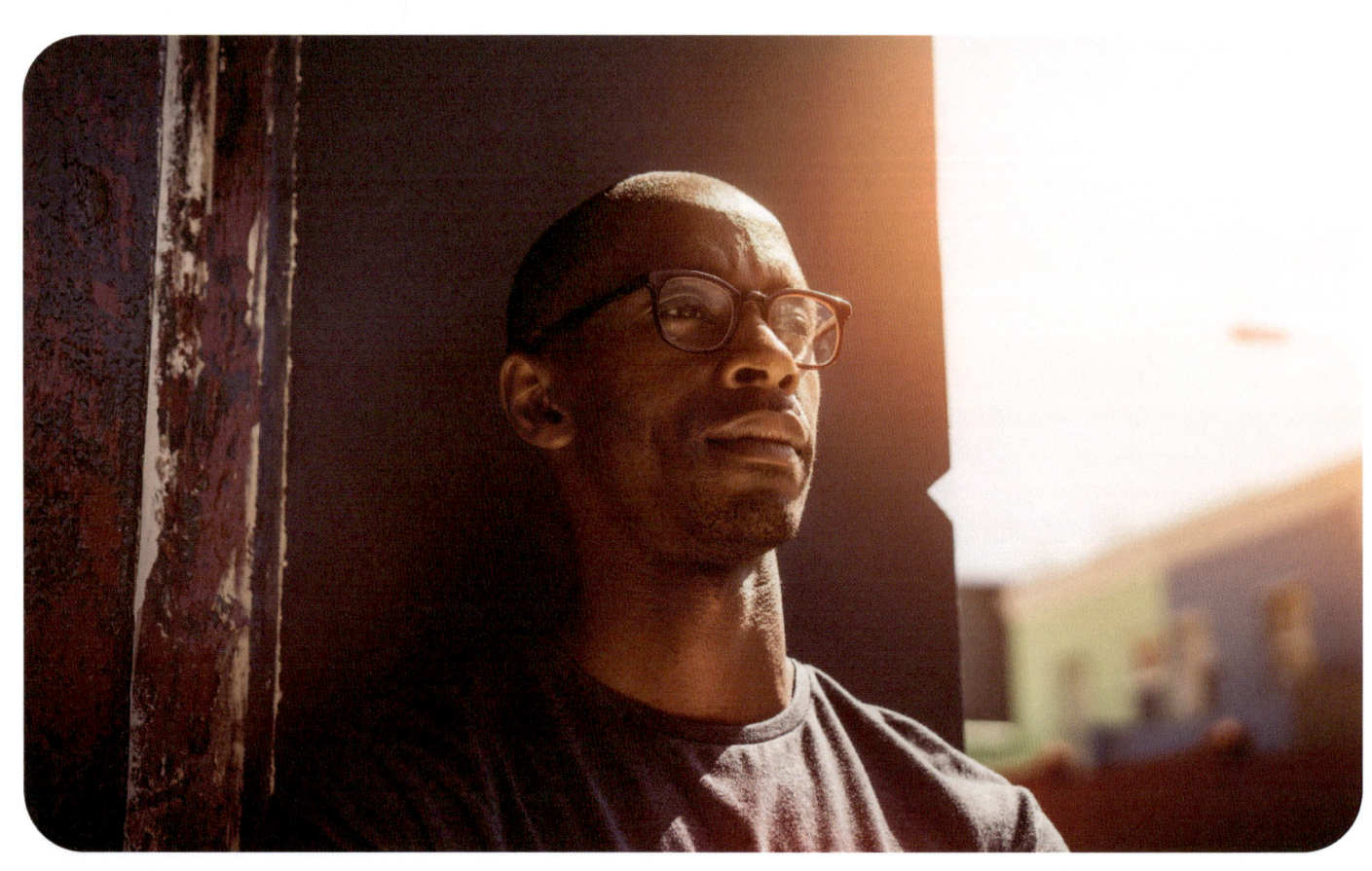

10 Making treatment decisions | It's your choice

It's important to be comfortable with the cancer treatment you choose. This choice starts with having an open and honest conversation with your doctor.

It's your choice

In shared decision-making, you and your doctors share information, discuss the options, and agree on a treatment plan. It starts with an open and honest conversation between you and your doctor.

Treatment decisions are very personal. What is important to you may not be important to someone else.

Some things that may play a role in your decision-making:

- What you want and how that might differ from what others want
- Your religious and spiritual beliefs
- Your feelings about certain treatments like surgery or chemotherapy
- Your feelings about pain or side effects such as nausea and vomiting
- Cost of treatment, travel to treatment centers, and time away from school or work
- Quality of life and length of life
- How active you are and the activities that are important to you

Think about what you want from treatment. Discuss openly the risks and benefits of specific treatments and procedures. Weigh options and share concerns with your doctor. If you take the time to build a relationship with your doctor, it will help you feel supported when considering options and making treatment decisions.

Second opinion

It is normal to want to start treatment as soon as possible. While cancer can't be ignored, there is time to have another doctor review your test results and suggest a treatment plan. This is called getting a second opinion, and it's a normal part of cancer care. Even doctors get second opinions!

Things you can do to prepare:

- Check with your insurance company about its rules on second opinions. There may be out-of-pocket costs to see doctors who are not part of your insurance plan.
- Make plans to have copies of all your records sent to the doctor you will see for your second opinion.

Support groups

Many people diagnosed with cancer find support groups to be helpful. Support groups often include people at different stages of treatment. Some people may be newly diagnosed, while others may be finished with treatment. If your hospital or community doesn't have support groups for people with cancer, check out the websites listed in this book.

Questions to ask your doctors

Possible questions to ask your doctors are listed on the following pages. Feel free to use these questions or come up with your own. Be clear about your goals for treatment and find out what to expect from treatment.

10 Making treatment decisions | Questions to ask your doctors

Questions to ask about testing and staging

1. What type of cancer do I have? What is the cancer stage? What does this mean?

2. Is it in my blood? Lymph nodes? Other organs?

3. When will I have a biopsy? What type of biopsy? What are the risks?

4. Is there a cancer center or hospital nearby that specializes in this type of cancer?

5. What tests are needed? What other tests do you recommend? Will I have any genetic or molecular tests?

6. What will you do to make me comfortable during testing?

7. How do I prepare for testing? How and where will the test be done?

8. How soon will I know the results and who will explain them to me?

9. Would you give me a copy of the pathology report and other test results?

10. Who will talk with me about the next steps? When?

11. Will treatment start before the test results are in?

12. Can my cancer be cured? If not, how well can treatment stop the cancer from growing?

10 Making treatment decisions | Questions to ask your doctors

Questions to ask about skin

1. Is this cancer contagious? Will it spread to people who touch me?

2. Should I avoid sharing clothes or towels? How often should I change or wash towels?

3. Can I use lotions or oils on my skin or hair other than what you give me? What about the best types of soap or shampoo? Hair dye? Makeup?

4. Is it better to wear long sleeves, pants, or cover the rash/lesions in some way? Or should I let them be exposed to the air as much as possible?

5. Should I take time to inspect my skin? If so, how often?

6. If I notice any changes in my skin whom should I call? When?

7. Will keeping a diary and photo journal help? What should I include in the diary? How often should I take photos?

8. Can I go out in the sun? Should I wear sunscreen? Long sleeves? Hat?

9. Are there any changes that I can make to my diet? Exercise?

10. What about stress? Will stress worsen my condition?

10 Making treatment decisions | Questions to ask your doctors

Questions to ask your doctors about their experience

1. What is your experience treating this type of cancer?

2. What is the experience of those on your team?

3. What types of cancer do you treat?

4. I would like to get a second opinion. Is there someone you recommend?

5. How many patients like me (of the same age, gender, race) have you treated?

6. Will you be consulting with experts to discuss my care? Whom will you consult?

7. How many procedures like the one you're suggesting have you done?

8. Is this treatment a major part of your practice?

9. How many of your patients have had complications? What were the complications?

10. Who will manage my day-to-day care?

10 Making treatment decisions | Questions to ask your doctors

Questions to ask about treatment

1. Which treatment do you recommend and why? Is this treatment a cure? What are the benefits and risks?

2. How long do I have to decide?

3. Will I have to go to the hospital or elsewhere for treatment? How often? How long is each visit? Will I have to stay overnight in the hospital or make travel plans?

4. Do I have a choice of when to begin treatment? Can I choose the days and times of treatment?

5. How much will the treatment hurt? What will you do to make me comfortable?

6. How much will this treatment cost? What does my insurance cover? Are there any programs to help pay for treatment?

7. What kind of treatment will I do at home? What can I do to prepare my home to ensure my safety or the safety of other family members in the household? What type of home care will I need?

8. Are there any life-threatening side effects of this treatment? How will these be monitored?

9. What should I expect from this treatment? How long will treatment last?

10. How do you know if treatment is working? How will I know if treatment is working?

11. What in particular should be avoided or taken with caution while receiving treatment?

12. What are the chances my cancer will return? Am I at risk for developing another kind of cancer, such as skin cancer?

10 Making treatment decisions | Questions to ask your doctors

Questions to ask about biopsies

1. What kind of biopsy will I have? Will I have more than one biopsy?

2. What types of tests will be done on the biopsy sample? What will you look for?

3. What will be removed during the biopsy?

4. How long will it take me to recover?

5. How much pain will I be in? What will be done to manage my pain?

6. What other side effects can I expect?

10 Making treatment decisions | Questions to ask your doctors

Questions to ask about radiation therapy

1. What type of radiation therapy (RT) will I have? How is this different from other types of RT?

2. What are the risks of this treatment?

3. What will you target?

4. What is the goal of this radiation treatment? Will RT be used with other therapies?

5. How many treatment sessions will I require? Can you do a shorter course of radiation?

6. Will I need someone to drive me home after treatment? What can I expect from treatment?

7. Do you offer this type of radiation here? If not, can you refer me to someone who does?

8. What side effects can I expect from radiation? How will these be treated?

10 Making treatment decisions | Questions to ask your doctors

Questions to ask about clinical trials

1. What clinical trials are available? Am I eligible for any of them? Why or why not?

2. What are the treatments used in the clinical trial?

3. What does the treatment do?

4. Has the treatment been used before? Has it been used for other types of cancer?

5. What are the risks and benefits of this treatment?

6. What side effects should I expect? How will the side effects be controlled?

7. How long will I be on the clinical trial?

8. Will I be able to get other treatment if this doesn't work?

9. How will you know the treatment is working?

10. Will the clinical trial cost me anything? If so, how much?

10 Making treatment decisions | Questions to ask your doctors

Questions to ask about stem cell transplants

1. How do you find a donor?

2. How long will I have to wait for a stem cell transplant (SCT)?

3. What do I need to do to prepare? What should I expect? What will you do to prepare?

4. What are the risks to myself and/or the donor?

5. How will the transplant affect my prognosis? Can cancer return after an SCT?

6. How will a transplant affect the quality and length of my life?

7. How long should I expect to be in the hospital?

8. How will I feel before, during, and after the transplant?

9. How many SCTs has this center done for those with this type of cancer?

10. What side effects may occur after an SCT?

11. Is radiation treatment included with an SCT?

12. Will I have more than one SCT?

10 Making treatment decisions | Questions to ask your doctors

Questions to ask about side effects

1. What are the side effects of treatment?

2. How long will these side effects last? Do any side effects lessen or worsen in severity over time?

3. What side effects should I watch for? What side effects are expected and which are life threatening?

4. When should I call the doctor? Can I text?

5. What medicines can I take to prevent or relieve side effects?

6. What can I do to help with pain and other side effects?

7. Will you stop treatment or change treatment if there are side effects? What do you look for?

8. What can I do to lessen or prevent side effects? What will you do?

9. What side effects are life-long and irreversible even after completing treatment?

10. What medicines may worsen side effects of treatment?

10 Making treatment decisions | Questions to ask your doctors

Questions to ask about survivorship and late effects

1. What happens after treatment?

2. What are the chances cancer will return or I will get another type of cancer?

3. Who do I see for follow-up care? How often? For how many years?

4. What should I do if I have trouble paying for follow-up visits and tests?

5. What tests will I have to monitor my health?

6. What late effects are caused by this treatment? How will these be screened?

7. I am looking for a survivor support group. What support groups or other resources can you recommend?

8. What happens if I move after treatment and have to change doctors? Will you help me find a doctor?

10 Making treatment decisions | Resources

Resources

American Academy of Dermatology Association (AADA)
aad.org/public

American Cancer Society (ACS)
Cancer.org

Cancer Hope Network
Cancerhopenetwork.org

Cutaneous Lymphoma Foundation (CLF)
clfoundation.org

International Society for Cutaneous Lymphomas (ISCL)
cutaneouslymphoma.org

Leukemia & Lymphoma Society (LLS)
LLS.org/informationspecialists

Lymphoma Research Foundation
lymphoma.org/aboutlymphoma/nhl/cbcl

lymphoma.org/aboutlymphoma/nhl/ctcl

MedlinePlus
medlineplus.gov/genetics/condition/mycosis-fungoides

medlineplus.gov/genetics/condition/sezary-syndrome/

National Cancer Institute (NCI)
cancer.gov/types/lymphoma/patient/mycosis-fungoides-treatment-pdq

How monoclonal antibodies treat cancer

National Coalition for Cancer Survivorship
canceradvocacy.org/toolbox

National Organization for Rare Diseases (NORD)
rarediseases.org

The Skin of Color Society (SOCS)
skinofcolorsociety.org

VisualDx
skinsight.com

Words to know

biopsy
The removal of a sample of tissue for testing.

blood tumor burden
The amount of cancerous cells in the blood.

body surface area (BSA)
The total surface area of the human body calculated using weight and height. Different than body mass index (BMI).

chemotherapy
Drugs that kill fast-growing cells, including cancer cells and normal cells.

clinical trial
A study of how safe and helpful tests and treatments are for people.

complete blood count (CBC)
A lab test that includes the number of blood cells.

complete response (CR)
No signs of cancer after treatment.

dermatologist
A doctor who specializes in the diagnosis and treatment of skin diseases.

external beam radiation therapy (EBRT)
A cancer treatment with radiation received from a machine outside the body.

erythema
Reddening of the skin, usually in patches.

erythroderma
A severe inflammation of most of the body's skin surface. It can look like sunburn or large splotches.

gene
Coded instructions in cells for making new cells and controlling how cells behave.

histology
The structure of cells, tissue, and organs as viewed under a microscope.

imaging test
A test that makes pictures (images) of the insides of the body.

immune system
The body's natural defense against infection and disease.

immunohistochemistry (IHC)
A lab test of cancer cells to find specific cell traits involved in abnormal cell growth.

involved-site radiation therapy (ISRT)
Targets a specific area of skin. It can also be used to treat specific lymph nodes with cancer.

lymph
A clear fluid containing white blood cells.

lymph node
A small, bean-shaped, disease-fighting structure.

lymphadenopathy
Lymph nodes that are abnormal in size or consistency.

medical oncologist
A doctor who is an expert in cancer drugs.

pallor
Skin that is paler than usual.

palpable adenopathy
Lymph nodes that feel abnormal in size or consistency.

Words to know

papule
A small, solid, raised bump on the skin that might look like small pimples. Papules may be red, purple, brown, or pink.

partial response (PR)
Some signs of cancra remain after treatment.

patch
A flat, thin, pink or red skin lesion of any size.

pathologist
A doctor who is an expert in testing cells and tissue to find disease.

persistent
Cancer that remains or returns.

phototherapy
uses different ultraviolet (UV) light wavelengths to treat skin lesions or tumors.

plaque
A raised (elevated) or hardened (indurated) skin lesion of any size.

progression
The growth or spread of cancer after being tested or treated.

pruritus
Itchy feeling that makes you want to scratch your skin.

radiation oncologist
A doctor who's an expert in treating cancer with radiation.

radiation therapy (RT)
A treatment that uses high-energy rays or related approaches to kill cancer cells.

radiologist
A doctor who is an expert in imaging tests.

recurrence
The return of cancer after a cancer-free period.

relapse
The return or worsening of cancer after a period of improvement.

refractory
Cancer that does not respond to multiple treatments.

regression
A decrease in the size of a patch, plaque, or tumor or the amount of cancer in the body.

remission
There are minor or no signs of disease.

retinoids
Products related to vitamin A.

scale
When the outer layer of skin peels away in large pieces.

side effect
An unhealthy or unpleasant physical or emotional response to treatment.

skin-directed therapy
Treatment focused on the skin. Includes topical therapy, local radiation, and phototherapy.

skin disease burden
The amount of cancerous cells found in the skin.

supportive care
Health care that includes symptom relief but not cancer treatment. Also called palliative care or best supportive care.

systemic therapy
Treatment that works throughout the body.

targeted therapy
A drug treatment that targets and attacks specific cancer cells.

total skin electron beam therapy (TSEBT)
Treats the entire skin surface.

NCCN Contributors

This patient guide is based on the NCCN Clinical Practice Guidelines in Oncology (NCCN Guidelines®) for Primary Cutaneous Lymphomas, Version 1.2021. It was adapted, reviewed, and published with help from the following people:

Dorothy A. Shead, MS
Director, Patient Information Operations

Rachael Clarke
Senior Medical Copyeditor

Tanya Fischer, MEd, MSLIS
Medical Writer

Laura J. Hanisch, PsyD
Medical Writer/Patient Information Specialist

Stephanie Helbling, MPH, CHES®
Medical Writer

Susan Kidney
Graphic Design Specialist

John Murphy
Medical Writer

Erin Vidic, MA
Medical Writer

Kim Williams
Creative Services Manager

The NCCN Guidelines® for Primary Cutaneous Lymphomas, Version 1.2021, were developed by the following NCCN Panel Members:

*Steven M. Horwitz, MD/Chair
Memorial Sloan Kettering Cancer Center

*Stephen Ansell, MD, PhD/Vice-Chair
Mayo Clinic Cancer Center

Weiyun Z. Ai, MD, PhD
UCSF Helen Diller Family Comprehensive Cancer Center

Jeffrey Barnes, MD, PhD
Massachusetts General Hospital Cancer Center

Stefan K. Barta, MD, MRCP, MS
Abramson Cancer Center at the University of Pennsylvania

Mark W. Clemens, MD
The University of Texas MD Anderson Cancer Center

*Ahmet Dogan, MD, PhD
Memorial Sloan Kettering Cancer Center

Aaron M. Goodman, MD
UC San Diego Moores Cancer Center

Gaurav Goyal, MD
O'Neal Comprehensive Cancer Center at UAB

Joan Guitart, MD
Robert H. Lurie Comprehensive Cancer Center of Northwestern University

Ahmad Halwani, MD
Huntsman Cancer Institute at the University of Utah

Bradley M. Haverkos, MD, MPH, MS
University of Colorado Cancer Center

Richard T. Hoppe, MD
Stanford Cancer Institute

Eric Jacobsen, MD
Dana-Farber/Brigham and Women's Cancer Center

Deepa Jagadeesh, MD, MPH
Case Comprehensive Cancer Center/ University Hospitals Seidman Cancer Center and Cleveland Clinic Taussig Cancer Institute

Allison Jones
St. Jude Children's Research Hospital/ The University of Tennessee Health Science Center

*Youn H. Kim, MD
Stanford Cancer Institute

*Neha Mehta-Shah, MD
Siteman Cancer Center at Barnes-Jewish Hospital and Washington University School of Medicine

Elise A. Olsen, MD
Duke Cancer Institute

Barbara Pro, MD
Robert H. Lurie Comprehensive Cancer Center of Northwestern University

Saurabh A. Rajguru, MD
University of Wisconsin Carbone Cancer Center

Sima Rozati, MD, PhD
The Sidney Kimmel Comprehensive Cancer Center at Johns Hopkins

Jonathan Said, MD
UCLA Jonsson Comprehensive Cancer Center

Aaron Shaver, MD, PhD
Vanderbilt-Ingram Cancer Center

Andrei Shustov, MD
Fred Hutchinson Cancer Research Center/ Seattle Cancer Care Alliance

Lubomir Sokol, MD, PhD
Moffitt Cancer Center

Pallawi Torka, MD
Roswell Park Cancer Institute

Carlos Torres-Cabala, MD
The University of Texas MD Anderson Cancer Center

Ryan Wilcox, MD, PhD
University of Michigan Rogel Cancer Center

Basem M. William, MD
The Ohio State University Comprehensive Cancer Center - James Cancer Hospital and Solove Research Institute

*Jasmine Zain, MD
City of Hope National Medical Center

NCCN

Mary Dwyer, MS
Director, Guidelines Operations

Hema Sundar, PhD
Manager, Global Clinical Content

* Reviewed this patient guide. For disclosures, visit NCCN.org/about/disclosure.aspx.

NCCN Cancer Centers

Abramson Cancer Center
at the University of Pennsylvania
Philadelphia, Pennsylvania
800.789.7366 • pennmedicine.org/cancer

Fred & Pamela Buffett Cancer Center
Omaha, Nebraska
402.559.5600 • unmc.edu/cancercenter

Case Comprehensive Cancer Center/
University Hospitals Seidman Cancer
Center and Cleveland Clinic Taussig
Cancer Institute
Cleveland, Ohio
800.641.2422 • UH Seidman Cancer Center
uhhospitals.org/services/cancer-services
866.223.8100 • CC Taussig Cancer Institute
my.clevelandclinic.org/departments/cancer
216.844.8797 • Case CCC
case.edu/cancer

City of Hope National Medical Center
Los Angeles, California
800.826.4673 • cityofhope.org

Dana-Farber/Brigham and
Women's Cancer Center |
Massachusetts General Hospital
Cancer Center
Boston, Massachusetts
617.732.5500
youhaveus.org
617.726.5130
massgeneral.org/cancer-center

Duke Cancer Institute
Durham, North Carolina
888.275.3853 • dukecancerinstitute.org

Fox Chase Cancer Center
Philadelphia, Pennsylvania
888.369.2427 • foxchase.org

Huntsman Cancer Institute
at the University of Utah
Salt Lake City, Utah
800.824.2073
huntsmancancer.org

Fred Hutchinson Cancer
Research Center/Seattle
Cancer Care Alliance
Seattle, Washington
206.606.7222 • seattlecca.org
206.667.5000 • fredhutch.org

The Sidney Kimmel Comprehensive
Cancer Center at Johns Hopkins
Baltimore, Maryland
410.955.8964
www.hopkinskimmelcancercenter.org

Robert H. Lurie Comprehensive
Cancer Center of Northwestern
University
Chicago, Illinois
866.587.4322 • cancer.northwestern.edu

Mayo Clinic Cancer Center
Phoenix/Scottsdale, Arizona
Jacksonville, Florida
Rochester, Minnesota
480.301.8000 • Arizona
904.953.0853 • Florida
507.538.3270 • Minnesota
mayoclinic.org/cancercenter

Memorial Sloan Kettering
Cancer Center
New York, New York
800.525.2225 • mskcc.org

Moffitt Cancer Center
Tampa, Florida
888.663.3488 • moffitt.org

The Ohio State University
Comprehensive Cancer Center -
James Cancer Hospital and
Solove Research Institute
Columbus, Ohio
800.293.5066 • cancer.osu.edu

O'Neal Comprehensive
Cancer Center at UAB
Birmingham, Alabama
800.822.0933 • uab.edu/onealcancercenter

Roswell Park Comprehensive
Cancer Center
Buffalo, New York
877.275.7724 • roswellpark.org

Siteman Cancer Center at Barnes-
Jewish Hospital and Washington
University School of Medicine
St. Louis, Missouri
800.600.3606 • siteman.wustl.edu

St. Jude Children's Research Hospital/
The University of Tennessee
Health Science Center
Memphis, Tennessee
866.278.5833 • stjude.org
901.448.5500 • uthsc.edu

Stanford Cancer Institute
Stanford, California
877.668.7535 • cancer.stanford.edu

UC San Diego Moores Cancer Center
La Jolla, California
858.822.6100 • cancer.ucsd.edu

UCLA Jonsson
Comprehensive Cancer Center
Los Angeles, California
310.825.5268 • cancer.ucla.edu

UCSF Helen Diller Family
Comprehensive Cancer Center
San Francisco, California
800.689.8273 • cancer.ucsf.edu

University of Colorado Cancer Center
Aurora, Colorado
720.848.0300 • coloradocancercenter.org

University of Michigan
Rogel Cancer Center
Ann Arbor, Michigan
800.865.1125 • rogelcancercenter.org

The University of Texas
MD Anderson Cancer Center
Houston, Texas
844.269.5922 • mdanderson.org

University of Wisconsin
Carbone Cancer Center
Madison, Wisconsin
608.265.1700 • uwhealth.org/cancer

UT Southwestern Simmons
Comprehensive Cancer Center
Dallas, Texas
214.648.3111 • utsouthwestern.edu/simmons

Vanderbilt-Ingram Cancer Center
Nashville, Tennessee
877.936.8422 • vicc.org

Yale Cancer Center/
Smilow Cancer Hospital
New Haven, Connecticut
855.4.SMILOW • yalecancercenter.org

Index

B cell (or B lymphocyte) 5

biomarkers 23–24

biopsy 21–22

body surface area (BSA) 17, 26

chemotherapy 35

clinical trials 36

clonal *TCR* gene rearrangements 24

cutaneous T-cell lymphoma (CTCL) 6

electron beam radiation therapy (EBRT) 34

erythroderma 18, 61

immunotherapy 35

involved-site radiation therapy (ISRT) 34

local therapy 32–33

lymph node 7, 27

lymphocytes 5

mycosis fungoides (MF) 10

phototherapy 33

primary cutaneous lymphoma (PCL) 9

radiation therapy (RT) 34

retinoids 35

Sézary syndrome (SS) 11, 61–62

skin-directed therapy 32–33

skin exam 17–18

staging 25–28

stem cell transplant (SCT) 37–38

supportive care 38

systemic category A (SYST-CAT A) 43, 53

systemic category B (SYST-CAT B) 43, 53

T cell (or T lymphocyte) 5

targeted therapy 35

topical therapy 32–33

total skin electron beam therapy (TSEBT) 34

visceral disease 64

Printed in Poland
by Amazon Fulfillment
Poland Sp. z o.o., Wrocław